COLLINS GEM
ANTIQUE MARKS

a mine of information

C000088140

COLLINS GEM
CRICKET

a mine of information

COLLINS GEM
DIETING

FAT

a mine of information

COLLINS GEM
DOGS

a mine of information

COLLINS GEM
FIRST AID

a mine of information

COLLINS GEM
INTERNET

www

@

Connect

a mine of information

COLLINS GEM
PREDICTING

a mine of information

COLLINS GEM
Ready
REFERENCE

a mine of information

COLLINS GEM
SHARKS

a mine of information

COLLINS GEM
WHALES & DOLPHINS

a mine of information

COLLINS GEM
WHISKY

a mine of information

COLLINS GEM
WORD PROCESSING

a mine of information

COLLINS GEM
Your PC

a mine of information

COLLINS GEM

MASSAGE

Roni Jay

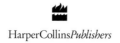

HarperCollins*Publishers*

Roni Jay is a professional writer and editor with a special interest in mind, body and spirit subjects.

HarperCollins Publishers
Westerhill Road, Bishopbriggs, Glasgow G64 2QT

Devised and created by The Printer's Devil, Glasgow

First published 2000

Reprint 10 9 8 7 6 5 4 3 2 1 0

Photography and art direction by PS5 Limited
With grateful thanks to Debs and Samantha

ISBN 0 00 472469 0

Printed in Italy by Amadeus S.p.A.

CONTENTS

These numbers which appear on the pictures refer the reader to corresponding numbered instructions in the text.

NOTE

While massage brings undoubted therapeutic benefits, there are a variety of circumstances when it is not recommended for particular individuals. Readers are advised to pay particular attention to the warnings given throughout the text and should consult with their own doctor if they have any doubts. The publishers do not accept responsibility for any problems arising from the misapplication of any techniques described in this book.

WHAT IS MASSAGE?

The word 'massage' originally comes from a Portuguese word meaning 'to knead'. Put simply, massage is the practice of rubbing or kneading parts of the body as a means of improving health. Generally, oils are used to help the hands glide over the skin; these are often scented for the therapeutic effects of the scent itself.

Massage is emotionally nourishing and soothing, and can be adapted to be either sedative or stimulating. As a sedative, it treats nervous problems such as headaches and insomnia, tension and emotional stress. As a stimulant, it can invigorate the system to alleviate fatigue and lethargy. Research indicates that giving and receiving a massage, can significantly reduce stress levels.

Benefits of Massage

Massage is far more than an emotionally therapeutic exercise. It also has numerous physical benefits, and can be used to treat all sorts of physical disorders:

Digestive disorders Massage can improve the action of the colon, strengthening the muscles of the intestines and the abdomen, and relieving constipation. It helps to get the digestive juices flowing, and helps the system to absorb food after it has been digested.

Kidney problems Kidney function can be improved through massage to help eliminate waste products and toxins, and reduce fluid retention.

Reproductive problems Back and abdominal massage can help to treat period cramps, irregular periods, PMS and the symptoms of the menopause.

Respiratory disorders Regular massage increases lung activity, leading to slower, deeper breathing. Certain movements can also help expel mucus from the lungs.

Lymphatic problems As the flow of lymph is stimulated, toxins are eliminated more efficiently. Swelling around injuries is also dispersed by this process, preventing adhesions from forming. (Adhesions are caused when the fluid in a swelling is not moved, but becomes sticky and adheres to the surrounding tissues restricting movement in the affected joint.)

Circulatory disorders Massage eases the pressure on the blood vessels, speeding up the flow of blood through the system. This helps with poor circulation and strengthens the heartbeat. It can therefore help treat cardiac problems, and reduce blood pressure and heart rate.

Muscular problems Massage can be adapted according to need. Movements which relax and stretch the muscles ease cramp and physical tension, and can break down scar tissue and help eliminate toxins. Contracting the muscles through massage improves muscle tone. Stiffness as a result of overactivity can be eased with movements which relax and contract the muscle by turns.

Skeletal problems Bones are not affected directly by massage but they can benefit indirectly. Improved blood and lymph circulation leads to better nutrition for bones, and massage gives relief to painful joint conditions such as arthritis.

Skin problems Massage stimulates glands in the skin, and improves its texture, tone and condition.

Despite its many curative properties, massage is generally preferred as a preventative treatment, simply because prevention is better than cure. Regular massage – which has long been the practice in many Eastern countries – can significantly improve overall health as well as emotional wellbeing.

THERAPEUTIC TREATMENT

Although many professionals offer experienced massage, it is perfectly possible to learn the skills for yourself. If you practise each movement as you learn it, and gradually add more to your repertoire, you can soon learn to give a skilled and beneficial massage.

The simple act of touching another person is hugely therapeutic in itself. We all know that babies need touching and caressing – according to research, most infants choose comforting physical contact in preference to food – and as we grow older we still need touch to soothe and comfort us. However, we tend to touch each other less as adults, which is one reason why massage is so valuable, as a tool for giving us back the physical contact we need emotionally.

An Ancient Art

Massage is the oldest physical medicine of all. It was certainly in use in China five thousand years ago, as it is referred to in the *Nei Ching*, the medical text written by the Yellow Emperor. In Egypt, wall paintings depict hand and foot massage as early as 2330 BC. And in India the *Ayurveda*, which dates from around 1800 BC, recommends rubbing the body to help it heal itself. In China, for example, there are still many regional styles of massage (it tends to be slow in the warm south, and vigorous in the colder north). Massage was an everyday part of life in the East, which has continued to the modern day in many places.

The Greeks and Romans knew a good deal more about human anatomy than many of their predecessors, and were great believers in the therapeutic and healing powers of massage. Socrates, Plato and Herodotus all made mention of massage and its benefits, and it is even mentioned in Homer's Odyssey as a restorative for exhausted soldiers. The Greek physician Asclepiades used a combination of massage and exercise for his patients, and the Roman naturalist Pliny had regular massage to treat his asthma. Julius

THE FATHER OF MEDICINE

The Greek physician Hippocrates, known as the father of modern medicine, wrote in the early fifth century BC: rubbing can bind a joint that is too loose, and loosen a joint that is too stiff. He recommended that all physicians should be trained in massage. He also recorded that 'rubbing up' was more effective than 'rubbing down' on the limbs, although with his incomplete understanding of the circulatory system he would not have known the reason for this.

Caesar was treated on a daily basis for neuralgia and headaches with massage and pinching.

When the Roman Empire collapsed, the practice of massage seems to have disappeared from Europe with it. The Christian church disapproved of such physical pleasures, being more focused on the health of the soul than of the body, so it took a long time for massage to reappear. The next recorded use of it is in the 16th century, following the Renaissance. Physical health was once again as important as it had been to the Romans, and many physicians began to use massage. One of the most influential of these physicians was the French doctor Ambrose Paré, who became the physician to four French kings.

Swedish Massage

The standard type of massage used in Europe is Swedish massage, which has been popular for nearly two hundred years. The strokes we use today were developed by the Swede Per Henrik Ling (*see below*), and we still use many of the French terms he gave to them.

THE BIRTH OF SWEDISH MASSAGE

Per Henrik Ling was born in 1776 in Sweden. He was originally a gymnast who also developed a massage technique in the early 19th century which brought together his training in gymnastics with massage skills he had learnt in China. This technique became known as Swedish massage, and remains largely unchanged even today. This form of mas-

Per Henrik Ling

sage had spread through Europe and across to America by the end of the 19th century. Societies of trained therapists were formed; in Britain the main society changed its name in 1934 to the Chartered Society of Physiotherapists.

After a while, the appeal of massage waned again, eclipsed by modern technological treatments, and by the fact that an effective massage session takes a good half an hour at least, and most physiotherapists simply don't have time for this.

But in the 1960s and '70s public opinion shifted once more, and many people were drawn to natural therapies without the use of drugs. This is still a prevailing view, and nowadays there is a demand for holistic treatments such as massage, which treat the mind, body and spirit together, just as massage has always been done in the East.

BODY POSITION

A Swedish massage is traditionally given on a massage couch, and you should keep your back straight while you are giving the massage, using your own body weight to create deep pressure. Swedish massage generally begins with the recipient lying on their back while you massage their feet and legs, then their hands and arms, followed by their abdomen and then their chest. Finally they turn over so you can massage their back.

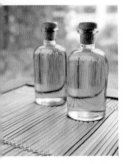

OILS

Oil is generally used in a
Swedish massage to help your
hands glide over the skin. Use
a basic carrier oil such as:

- Grapeseed oil
- Sweet almond oil
- Soya oil
- Sunflower oil
- Apricot kernel oil

All these carrier oils are rich
in vitamins and minerals, and will help to moisturise
the skin as well as easing the massage. You can add a
few drops of essential oil to your carrier oil if you
wish.

You may also add a specialist carrier oil to create a
more nourishing and moisturising blend. If you want
to do this, mix your basic carrier in a proportion of
about 5:1 with an oil such as wheatgerm, avocado,
sesame or jojoba.

NUT ALLERGY

If the person you are massaging has a nut allergy,
you must avoid using a nut-derived oil. Ask *before*
you begin massaging if you are unsure and always
have a variety of oils to hand just in case.

HAND MOVEMENTS

Strokes

Massage employs a range of hand movements, each of which has a particular function: some relax, some stimulate, some stretch, some warm up and so on. Once you are skilled in massage you will know exactly which type of movement to use and when. Although the movements should flow smoothly into one another, they are very distinct.

Swedish massage still uses the names for these movements that Per Henrik Ling (*see p. 10*) gave them nearly two hundred years ago. Understanding how to use these movements, and knowing when each is appropriate, is central to learning massage.

CORE STROKES IN SWEDISH MASSAGE

Effleurage gentle stroking which is given at the beginning and end of the massage

Petrissage this involves squeezing the muscles, and includes kneading

Superficial strokes derived from petrissage, these are only skin deep

Percussion this stimulates the body towards the end of the treatment

---

EFFLEURAGE

Effleurage is a very gentle and soothing stroke. If you are massaging with oil it helps to spread the oil evenly over the skin. Although the stroke is very light, it stimulates the nerve endings in the part of the body being touched, and creates awareness in the surface muscles and skin.

Effleurage should be used at the beginning of any treatment to attune the body to the massage, and at the end of the treatment to leave the body alert but

Effleurage

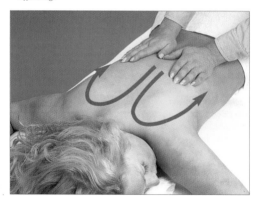

relaxed. It is also a useful stroke to use to ease the flow from one movement to another during the massage.

The slower effleurage is, the more of a calming effect it has on your partner. It is very effective on its own for treating stress and emotional tension, and can relieve tension headaches and poor sleeping. Brisker effleurage will help to revive and stimulate someone who is tired and drained.

Effleurage is given with the palms of both hands, gliding gently but firmly over the skin. Apply continuous pressure as you slide your hands along the skin, and then return them in a circular movement to their starting position. If you are effleuraging the back, for example, sweep your hands up the spine and then down the sides of the chest before repeating the movement. (*See illustration opposite.*)

To effleurage narrower areas such as legs or arms, place one hand in front of the other on the skin. When you reach the end of the arm or leg, raise the first hand and replace it at the start position before lifting the other hand from the skin. This way, one or other of your hands is always in contact with your partner's skin. You can also use effleurage on the face; in this case, as with any other smaller area, you will need to use your fingertips rather than your whole hand. (*See illustration, p. 16.*)

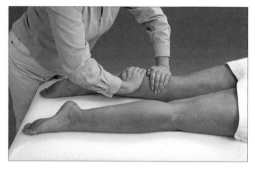

Effleurage on a narrow area

PETRISSAGE

This term derives from the French word meaning 'to knead', and is used to describe any movement which squeezes the muscles, such as kneading or wringing. The basic petrissage stroke entails taking hold of part of a muscle and squeezing it with your thumbs and fingers. By alternately squeezing and relaxing, you are emptying the blood and lymph vessels and then allowing them to refill. This increases the blood supply to the muscle (so don't worry if it looks a little red), and helps to speed up the elimination of toxins. It is useful after exercise to prevent the muscles getting stiff, and can help alleviate spasms and cramps. It also helps to break down fatty deposits around the buttocks, thighs

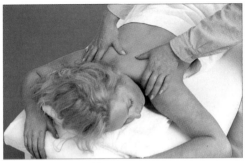

Petrissage on the shoulders

and shoulders. Petrissage works best on the legs, buttocks and shoulders.

To apply petrissage to the shoulders, squeeze along the top of the shoulders with the greatest pressure coming from the ball of your thumb, with your fingers resting more lightly. (*See illustration above.*)

To work on the inner thigh, ask your partner to lie on their back, and place a pillow under the knee. Hold the muscles inside the knee between your fingers and thumb, leaving space between the palm of your hand and the leg. Squeezing the muscle with alternate hands, stroke gently up the inner thigh and back down again. Gradually decrease the pressure as you

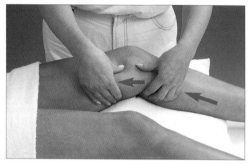

Petrissage on the legs

move up the thigh, and increase it again as you move back down. (*See illustration above.*)

KNEADING

This form of petrissage can be either calming or invigorating depending on how you use it. If it is slow and deep, it is the deepest stroke there is in Swedish massage, and it breaks down deep-seated tension in the muscle. Applied more vigorously it stimulates the circulation and revives the body. It is at its best on fleshy areas such as the buttocks, thighs and waist, and is also effective on the calves. It can be tiring for both of you, so alternate kneading with a few effleurage strokes if necessary.

WARNING

Never use kneading on the legs if there are broken
or varicose veins.

To knead, grasp the flesh with both hands and
squeeze with one hand pushing the flesh towards the
other hand. Then release and squeeze with the other
hand, pushing it back again. You can also knead less
fleshy areas, such as the neck, with your fingertips
only to release tension in the top layer of muscle. (*See
illustration below*)

Kneading

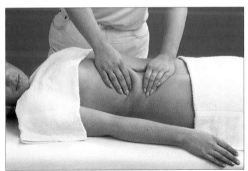

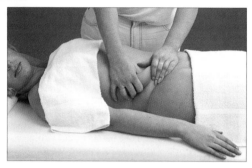

Wringing

WRINGING

This is a variation on kneading. Start as if for kneading, and then pull the flesh up and twist it into your other hand as if you were wringing out a cloth. Release and repeat back and forth from hand to hand. This is an extremely deep stroke which will release deep muscle tension. (*See illustration above.*)

SUPERFICIAL STROKES

These movements all derive from petrissage, but they are only skin deep. They work on the nervous system through the nerve endings close to the skin so that, although the strokes are gentle, they can still be deeply effective.

These superficial strokes are very useful for massaging injured areas, or for a relaxing aromatherapy massage. They help to loosen the tissues and boost the circulation, and are mildly stimulating.

CIRCLING

This is similar to effleurage, but the circles can be any size, and are generally formed with one hand on top of the other. You can apply very small circles with the fingertips only. This stroke is generally given to the back or buttocks. Place one hand on your partner's back or buttocks with the other hand over the top. Sweep your hands round by rotating your wrists in a circle keeping a constant light pressure. (*See illustration below.*)

Circling

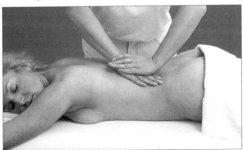

FANNING

This combines friction (*see p. 25*) and stretching (*see p. 32*), and is best used on large areas of muscle, such as on the back or the stomach. Brisk fanning warms the muscles up for aromatherapy, while slow fanning is very soothing, and can even be used to finish off a massage instead of the more usual effleurage.

Place the heel of one hand on your partner's back or stomach, allowing your fingers to fan out. Now rotate your hand applying steady pressure with the heel of your hand, and allow your fingers to trail behind. When your hand has rotated as far as it can, replace it

Fanning

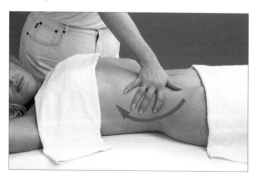

with your other hand, placing the heel a little higher up the body. Fan this hand back to the starting point, so that the fingers trail over the same area of the skin as the fingers of your first hand did. (*See illustration opposite.*)

ROLLING

This treatment should be given towards the end of the massage, when the skin is warm and relaxed. It is a treatment for the skin which improves its tone, circulation and drainage. It should not be painful. It works well where the skin is easy to pick up, such as across the shoulders and down the back.

Rolling

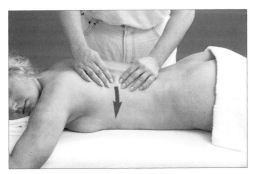

Gently gather up a fold of skin between your fingers and thumbs using both hands. Now move your fingers forwards a little, and then bring the thumbs up behind so that a wave of skin is brought along with them. 'Roll' this wave of skin to the edge of the shoulder or back in this way. You can repeat this movement all over the shoulders and back, working outwards from the middle down both sides. (*See illustration on p. 23.*)

PICKING UP

This stroke focuses on the skin, although it also treats the muscles beneath. It is used to tone the skin on broad areas of the body such as the stomach and back.

Place the thumb and fingertips of both hands on your partner's skin to start. Now with your left hand press inwards and slightly downwards as if you were gently pinching a lump of flesh. At the same time lift your right hand away from the skin with the fingers outstretched.

Now quickly reverse these positions – the right hand descends to pick up a fold of flesh while the left hand lifts and spreads out. Avoid pinching the skin as you do this. Keep repeating this brisk movement, increasing the speed and the depth of the movement, for about fifteen or twenty seconds at a time. (*See illustration opposite.*)

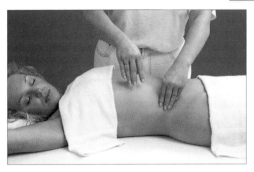

Picking up

FRICTION

Friction is clearly a warming stroke, but it also helps to loosen muscles, break down knots and the adhesions that can follow injury, and break down fatty tissue. You can apply friction with the side of your hands, a loose fist or with your fingers spread out, depending on which part of the body you are working on. On hairy parts of the body, make sure you apply a little oil before you begin.

To apply friction to the back of the thigh, place the edges of your hands parallel to each other. Move them quickly backwards and forwards in opposite directions, in contact with the thigh, and gradually move the process up and down the thigh. Do this in bursts of fifteen to thirty seconds. (*See illustration below.*)

To apply friction to the chest and back, spread your hand out loosely against the skin. Using large side-to-side wrist movements, rub the skin so that the heel of your hand remains roughly stationary but the fingers brush the skin. Move your hand up and down the chest or back. A similar action, but with a smaller movement and a loose fist, can be used to apply friction to the shoulders. (*See illustration opposite.*)

This is not a deep muscle treatment, but it should reach the muscles below the skin and not the skin alone. Do not overheat the skin or it will become

Friction applied to the thigh

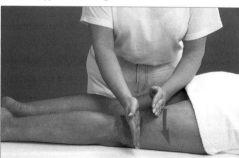

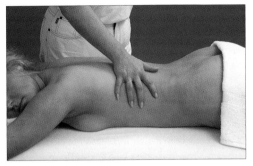

Friction applied to the back

painful. And watch your own posture or you will
overtense your shoulders.

RAKING

This stroke works well on the back and is very relaxing, despite being a vigorous movement. It is very
warming and is effective on tired or tense muscles.

Place your hands on your partner's back, positioning
them like rakes, with the fingers rigid. Draw them
firmly and briskly across the back. When you reach
the end of the stroke, return your hands to the starting position and keep repeating it for about ten seconds. As an alternative, you can move your hands

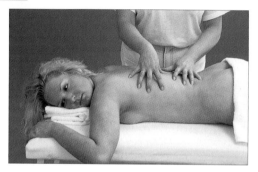

Raking

alternately backward and forward, instead of moving them together. (*See illustration above.*)

PUMMELLING

This stroke does not actually involve striking your partner's body – in fact, your hands never lose contact with their skin. The action entails shaking your hands so as to vibrate the muscles in your partner's body. It works well as an alternative to picking up (*see p. 24*), on parts of the body where picking up doesn't work, such as the legs and shoulders.

To pummel the top of the thigh, make a fist with each hand, and place the edges of the fists against the out-

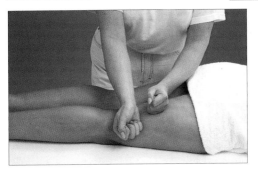

Pummelling

side of the thigh. Keep one fist still and roll the other
back a little from the wrist. Now roll the second fist
back as you return the first to its starting position.
Continue this forward and backward rolling with both
hands at speed for about ten to fifteen seconds. (*See
illustration above.*)

THUMBING

Thumbing is a useful stroke to apply to specific areas
where the muscles are tense or there are old adhesions. It involves twisting the skin over the muscle,
and should be painless even on a tense area of the
body. You need to keep your thumbs straight, and use
sufficient pressure to indent the skin slightly.

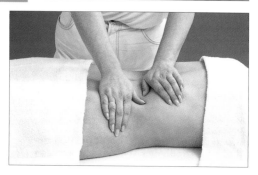

Thumbing

Place your thumbs and fingertips on your partner, with your fingers together and your thumbs a little way apart from each other. Slide your left thumb in front of your right, and your right thumb behind your left. Move your thumbs back and forth in little semi-circles like this, getting faster as you go, for about fifteen seconds. Shift your original hand position slightly and then repeat. *(See illustration above.)*

PRESSING

This stroke works well for applying pressure down the sides of the back. Your hands should be crossed over to help you apply even pressure. Ask your partner to breathe out as you start to press, and breathe in as you return your hands to the starting position. Don't make direct contact with the neck or the base of the spine.

Place your hands flat on the lower back, with the wrists crossed over and the heels of your hands touching each other. Your hands should rest either side of the spine, not on it. Press firmly so that your hands slide around your partner's waist, still pressing. Check that they have exhaled and then bring your hands back the same way, under slightly less pressure. Repeat this movement three times and then move up the back gradually until you reach the shoulders. (*See illustration below.*)

Pressing

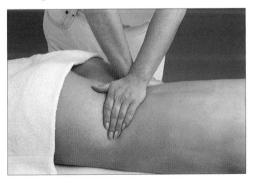

STRETCHING

This stroke benefits the skin and increases its elasticity. It involves moving the skin across the muscles that lie beneath it, and it works particularly well on the back.

Place your hands beside each other, palm down, a little way apart. Pressing firmly but not deeply, slide them forward and back in opposite directions, pulling the skin with them. Repeat the movement in reverse. Continue back and forth five times, and then repeat the stroke over the whole of the back. *(See illustration below.)*

Stretching

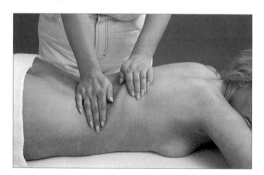

> ## WARNING
>
> **Never** use percussion strokes on the kidneys and spine, bony areas, bruises or broken veins

PERCUSSION

Percussion movements are designed to stimulate and invigorate. They boost the circulation, improve muscle and skin tone, and help bring your partner back from deep relaxation. There are several rules for percussion movements; see the coloured panels on this page.

> ## PERCUSSION MOVEMENTS
>
> Percussion movements should be:
>
> * light so as not to hurt your partner
>
> * moved around an area, not focused on one spot
>
> * built up to a crescendo over about thirty seconds, from slow to very fast, and then stopped suddenly
>
> * generated by wrist action rather than by moving your hands or fingers

BEATING

This is the deepest percussion stroke, ideal for using on well-muscled areas of the body such as the legs, buttocks and upper arms. It stimulates deep into the muscle.

Form your hands into loose fists, with the wrists relaxed. Now use your hands alternately to strike the body lightly, flicking each fist away from the body as soon as it touches the skin. Gradually build up speed before stopping suddenly, and avoid hitting any bones. *(See illustration below.)*

Beating

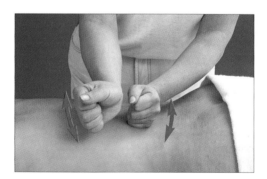

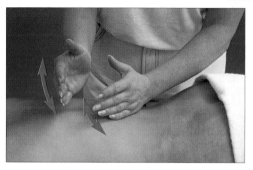

Hacking

HACKING

This is very similar to beating, except that you use the sides of your open hands. You can use it on any part of the body suitable for percussion strokes apart from the face. The most difficult thing about using this stroke is maintaining even pressure with both hands.

Keep your hands flat but relaxed, and lay the sides of them on your partner's body. Focus on the upward movement, flicking each hand away from the skin as soon as it touches it. Your relaxed fingers should knock against each other as you hack. *(See illustration above.)*

CUPPING

This stroke works on the larger muscles of the body such as those of the back and the buttocks. It is also useful, however, on the ribcage to loosen any congestion. You need to make a watertight cup with your hands and, once again, move your hands up and down in quick succession against the body.

Strike the body as for other percussion strokes, but this time with your hands firmly cupped. This should create a hollow sound as each hand makes contact with the skin. You don't need to raise your hands very far from your partner's body on each stroke. *(See illustration below.)*

Cupping

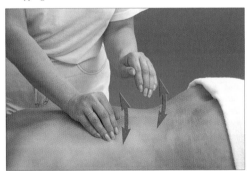

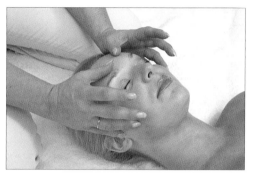

Tapotement

TAPOTEMENT

This light tapping is generally used on the face, although it is also suitable for any other areas that are delicate. It is the gentlest form of percussion, and relaxes the body generally while also stimulating the muscles of the face. It is the ideal way to finish a facial massage.

Hold your hands lightly open and rhythmically tap or drum the fingers of both hands against the skin. Be especially gentle when working around the eyes and the tip of the nose, but don't forget to include the ears. Work from the centre along the underside of the chin, then over the cheeks and temples, and finally across the forehead and then the ears. *(See illustration on p. 37.)*

PREPARATION

Before you can begin to give a massage, you need to prepare. Massage must be given in the right position and place; if your partner isn't comfortable the massage will be less effective.

And don't forget about yourself. If your posture is wrong you could end up needing a massage yourself by the end of the session. You also need to prepare your hands so that they don't become cramped and painful as you give the massage.

CHOOSING THE PLACE

You should always give a massage in a warm, comfortable room, in a relaxed atmosphere. Close the door and put the answerphone on, and dim the lights. A bedroom or sitting room is fine; choose somewhere which will be warm for your partner even when they have removed most of their clothes, and where you are not going to be interrupted.

You might want to play some relaxing music in the background while you massage, and perhaps burn some incense or essential oil.

If you have the choice, it's better to use a room decorated in soft pastel shades, since these are the

most relaxing colours. In any case, avoid rooms
decorated in strong bright colours such as reds and
oranges.

GETTING COMFORTABLE

You need a firm but comfortable flat surface to give a
massage. This means that any but the hardest beds are
not ideal. However you can use the floor or a table if
you don't have a professional couch. The one

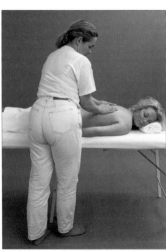

drawback to using the floor is that you are likely to injure yourself if you use any vigorous techniques. Both the floor and a table will need some padding to make them comfortable – a futon mattress, a folded quilt or two or three blankets.

While your partner is lying on their back, they will generally need a small pillow under their knees. This helps to relax the lower back, stomach and legs. A folded towel under the head will keep their spine straight.

When your partner is lying face down, as you work on their back, neck or the backs of the legs, put a small pillow under the ankles and another under the stomach. Place the folded towel under the upper chest to relax the neck.

GETTING YOUR EQUIPMENT READY

Before you begin your massage you will need:

- 2 pillows
- plenty of clean, warm towels
- oil (*see p. 12*)

A Swedish massage is generally given with no clothes on; however if this makes you or your partner feel uncomfortable, suggest they leave their underwear on. You will need towels to cover any exposed parts of your partner, from the chest to the knees, which you are not working on. Unless the room is very warm, your partner will appreciate it if you can keep the towels somewhere warm such as on a radiator or heated rail until you use them. Remember that someone lying very still with almost no clothes on will get cold easily; you, on the other hand, are dressed and actively giving the massage.

You will also need to warm the oil before you put it on your partner's skin. This is generally done by warming it in your hands for a few moments first.

GETTING YOURSELF READY

You will become tired and develop backache if you don't practise good posture during the massage. As

FOR YOUR AND YOUR PARTNER'S HEALTH AND COMFORT

- Wear loose, comfortable clothes. You needn't wear shoes if you are more comfortable without.

- Keep your hair well out of the way of your partner; if it is long, tie it back.

- Wash your hands thoroughly before and after a massage.

RULES FOR GOOD POSTURE

- Always stand close to your partner while massaging them.

- Face the part of the body you are working on.

- Keep your back straight and relaxed at all times.

- Distribute your weight evenly between your feet. If necessary, shift the weight from one foot to the other.

- If you are giving a deep massage, use your body weight to apply pressure, not muscle force.

- Do not give a massage while kneeling if you can avoid it, since you are likely to strain your back.

well as the obvious disadvantage to you, this will also take your concentration away from your partner. There are some basic guidelines for good posture; the Rules For Good Posture above shows these, and the illustration on page 40 shows the correct posture for giving a massage.

Your state of mind is also important. Make sure you

are calm and relaxed before you begin the treatment. You might like to do a little meditating or at least breathing exercises to relax you; or perhaps some gentle stretching if you find physical exercise relaxing. You will also need to exercise your hands in preparation; some hand exercises are outlined on the pages that follow.

HAND EXERCISES

Your hands are your most important piece of equipment, and they need to be strong, relaxed and flexible. Regular hand exercises will help you to achieve this.

1 Put the palms of your hands together in front of you in a praying position. Now raise your elbows so that your palms separate, and press your fingers together for a count of ten.

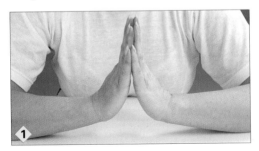

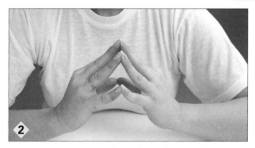

2 Next, open your hands so that only your fingertips are touching; press these together for a further count of ten. Return to the starting position and repeat five times.

3 Hold your hands in front of you in a praying position again. Now rotate your wrists and forearms

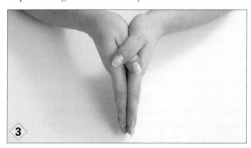

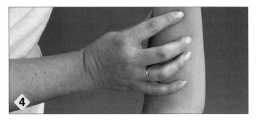

so that the tips of your fingers touch your chest. Return to the starting position and repeat five times.

4 Drum your fingers up and down the lower half of your other arm for about twenty or thirty seconds. Speed up and slow down, and vary the pressure, as you do it. Repeat with the fingers of the other hand.

As well as routine exercising, always try to use these exercises before and after each massage you give.

UNDERLYING TECHNIQUES

The rhythm of repetitive movements is much of what makes a massage so relaxing and therapeutic. However, there are certain aspects of maintaining this rhythm which improve with practice. The easiest way

to learn massage is to try to master a few strokes or
steps at a time before you move on to the next batch.
But whichever strokes you are practising, there are
three underlying techniques of massage that you need
to grasp:

- Speed
- Pressure
- Continuity

SPEED

Most massage strokes can be given at any tempo from
very slow to vigorous. The slower a stroke is, the more
relaxing it will be, while the faster strokes are
stimulating. So you need to be able to vary the tempo
of the movements.

Begin the massage at the tempo you feel your partner
is at – if they are agitated, start with brisk, stimulating
strokes and gradually slow them down as your partner
relaxes; if they are lethargic, begin with deep, slow
strokes and speed up by degrees.

You need to be able to judge what kind of speed your
partner needs, by determining whether their overall
need is for stimulation or relaxation. You will still
want to move into a relaxing massage and finish with
a few brisk strokes to revive your partner, but you will
have to be sensitive to their frame of mind to ascertain
the general tempo of the overall massage.

PRESSURE

The lighter the pressure, the more relaxing the massage will be; however it will not be so effective at clearing tension and knotted muscles. So begin the massage with light pressure, but deepen it over the first few minutes. Use your body weight to increase the pressure. The pressure should not, however, be painful.

Some tender areas are bound to need work, but this should feel beneficial to your partner, not just unpleasant.

CONTINUITY

One of the most important aspects of massage is the continuous fluid movement which your partner experiences; it is important that you shouldn't stop, and you should never be out of contact with their skin for more than a split second. If you are moving round them to work on another part of their body, keep one hand in contact with them as you do so.

If you are still learning and can't remember the next movement, keep stroking your partner until you think of it. Gentle stroking, or effleurage (see p. 00), is a good way to link different stages of a massage.

EXTREME RESPONSES

Sometimes, your partner may be ticklish. This is a sign of tension, so the best cure is to relax the area. Use

slow, stroking movements with a flat hand to do this.
After a while, you may be able to massage without
tickling. If not, leave the area until another time.

At the opposite extreme, your partner may fall asleep
during the massage. Take this as a compliment; it is a
sign of deep relaxation. Just carry on with the massage,
and you should find it easier to get into the muscles.

When Not to Massage

There are certain conditions which make massage
painful, risky – either for you or your partner – or

DO NOT MASSAGE OVER OR NEAR THE FOLLOWING AREAS:

- Thrombo-phlebitis
- Varicose veins
- Recent scars
- Abdomen during early pregnancy
- Lumps
- Inflamed areas, such as housemaid's knee or any inflamed organ
- Unexplained discomfort or pain
- Recent injection sites, especially cortisone

DO NOT MASSAGE AT ALL IF THE PERSON:

- has suffered a serious injury in the previous 48 hours

- has a degenerative condition

- has had recent surgery

- is on major medication

- is currently being treated with a manipulative therapy such as osteopathy

- has a high temperature

- has an infectious skin condition (acne, psoriasis and eczema are not infectious)

even dangerous. On the following page are checklists of conditions with which you must take care.

Page 49 carries a list showing conditions where massage is contraindicated near the area affected.

On this page a list of more serious conditions, where you should not attempt to massage the person at all.

BODY MASSAGE

HOW TO GIVE A MASSAGE

Having mastered the basic techniques, you can now go on to give a full body massage. The numbered step-by-step pictures take you through the whole massage and are divided into sections according to the parts of the body. You don't have to give the entire set – you can miss out some parts and give more time to others.

TIMING A MASSAGE

A whole massage should last between an hour and an hour and a half. On occasions when you have less than an hour, you can simply leave out certain areas. However, a whole body massage of less than about half an hour isn't really worth having, since there isn't time for your partner to go through the relaxing and restimulating process for long enough to be beneficial. Where time is limited, it is generally more useful to focus on one or two parts of the body only. Just give a neck and shoulder massage, for example, or just a face massage (which relaxes the whole body).

Remember to begin and end every massage session with effleurage strokes.

Parts of the Body

The following steps give a complete massage for each
part of the body. When giving a whole body massage,
simply follow each of these sections one after another.

BACK AND SHOULDERS

It is traditional to begin a whole body massage with
the back, where the major postural muscles are. It also
one of the easiest areas to work on since it is the
largest, and is covered with large muscles (see p. 00).
A lot of tension can be stored in the back, and a back
massage is a very effective way to relax your partner.

GETTING READY

- Your partner should lie on their front with a
  pillow under the head and shoulders and one
  under the feet. They may also be comfortable
  with a third pillow under their stomach.

- Their arms should be at their sides, hanging
  over the edge of the couch or table, or bent with
  their hands by their head.

- Their head should be turned to whichever side is
  most comfortable for them, or their forehead
  should rest on their hands.

- Cover their buttocks and legs with a towel.

- If you use oil, apply it to your hands to warm it.

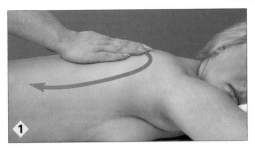

1 Place your hands at either side of the base of the spine. Effleurage the back with large, sweeping strokes either side of the spine from the base up to the shoulders, then more lightly down the sides of the back. Repeat this stroke several times, for about 30 seconds.

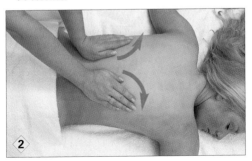

2 Place your hands either side of the base of the spine (not on it), with the heels of your hands closer together than the fingers. Effleurage in circles up and out to the sides, then down and back in. Work up the spine in this way until you reach the top.

3 Return to the same starting position, but this time with the heels of your hands either side of the spine and your fingers facing outwards. Apply petrissage by pressing the heels of your hands into the grooves either side of the spine and pushing them towards your fingers, which should remain in the same place and not slide round the edge of the back.

4 Working on one shoulder, pick up the muscle just below the armpit and knead by squeezing it. Now squeeze with the other hand just above the first, and set up a rhythmic kneading from one hand to the other for about 20 seconds.

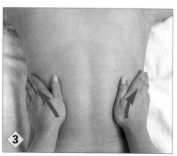

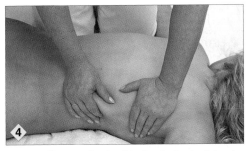

5 Now effleurage the shoulder by placing both hands on the shoulder blade and stroking firmly towards the arm, then circling back to the starting point. Use your body weight to apply firm pressure. Now repeat these last two steps on the other shoulder.

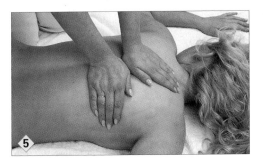

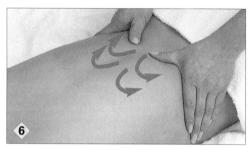

6 Place the balls of your thumbs either side of the spine (not on it) and apply friction up the spine by circling with your thumbs either side of the spine from the base to the neck. If you feel knots and nodules, work over the area for a little longer. The pressure should be fairly deep and slow, and will probably make your thumbs ache. Bring your hands back to the starting point with a light stroke down the back, and repeat the whole movement twice.

7 Now place your thumbs at the same starting point but this time glide them straight up either side of the spine to the neck, with firm pressure. Repeat this four times.

8 Using your left hand, petrissage along the top of the left shoulder working outwards, being careful not to pinch. Now do this on the right shoulder using the right hand. Repeat the sequence – left and right shoulders – four times.

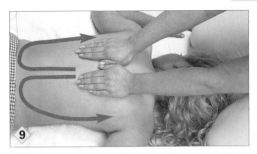

9 Keeping one hand on the centre of your partner's back, between the shoulder blades, move around to stand at your partner's head. Place your hands either side of the top of the spine and effleurage firmly down the back, leaning your body weight into the stroke. Bring your hands back more lightly up the sides of the back as far as the armpits, and then across the shoulder blades. Repeat four times.

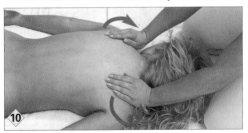

10 Glide your hands out so they are positioned round the top edge of the shoulders. Scoop your hands round in circles, pressing with the heels of your hands, and work in towards the neck. Repeat twice.

11 Place both hands on the same shoulder with your thumbs facing each other and lying lengthwise along the top of the shoulder. Lean your body weight into your thumbs and glide them along the shoulder muscle to the top of the arm. Repeat twice on this side, and then move to the other side.

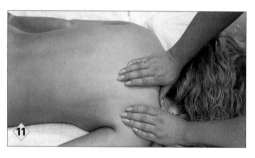

12 Perform the same movement again, but this time with one thumb on each side, close to the centre. Lean into the movement and glide the thumbs out towards the top of the shoulders. Repeat twice.

13 Now place your thumbs either side of the top of the spine, and the flats of your hands out to the sides.

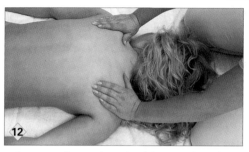

Petrissage down either side of the spine from the
neck to the base, pressing your thumbs firmly on
the muscles either side of the spine (not on it).
Work down and up the spine three times.

14 Keeping one hand on your partner's body, move
round to stand to one side of them. Use hacking on

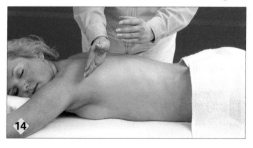

the whole of the upper back (avoiding direct contact with the spine). Begin slowly and build up speed over the tops of the shoulders, the edge of the chest and the rest of the upper back. Hack for 30 seconds and then stop abruptly.

15 Now use cupping to percuss the lower back and around the edge of the pelvis. Again, start slowly and build up speed, stopping after about 20 to 30 seconds. Listen for the hollow sound as the cupped hand strikes the body.

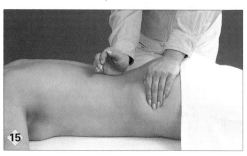

16 Repeat the effleurage from the beginning of the massage, as shown in step 1. Do this for about a minute, letting the strokes become lighter and lighter until your partner can barely feel them at all. Finally, bring the towel up to cover your partner's back.

BUTTOCKS AND LEGS

The buttocks and legs contain powerful muscles which support the weight of the body. Regular movement of these muscles helps the circulation and, in effect, the legs massage themselves up to a point when we move and walk. But tired legs and buttocks can lead to cramps and varicose veins, so a massage is valuable. Massaging the backs of the legs can help relieve pain in the lower back, as these two areas are often linked. The legs are always effleuraged upwards to stimulate the circulation.

GETTING READY

- Your partner should have a pillow under their feet when lying on their front.

- When they lie on their back, move the pillow underneath the knees.

- Cover their back and shoulders with one towel, and use another over the buttocks except when you are working on them.

- When massaging the legs, use a towel to cover the leg you are not working on.

- Do not use strong pressure over varicose veins.

- Do not use strong pressure on the back of the knee.

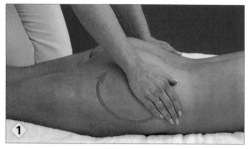

1 To massage the buttocks, begin by placing your
hands on either side of the lower back, fingers
pointing towards the side of the waist, and
effleuraging. Stroke down and around the sides of
the buttocks and then back up over the top to the
starting position. Repeat four times.

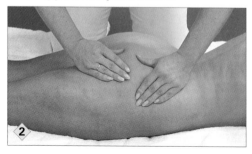

2 Stand to the side of your partner and work on the buttock furthest from you. Knead the buttock by picking up the muscle between the fingers and thumb of one hand and squeezing. As you release, squeeze the muscle just above this with the other hand. Squeezing your hands alternately, knead all over the buttock for about 30 seconds.

3 Place the heel of one hand at the top of the buttock. Push it down the side of the buttock to squeeze the muscle between the heel and the fingers. Repeat with the other hand. Do this four or five times, working down the buttock. Keep one hand on your partner's body, and move round to the other side. Repeat the last two steps on the other side.

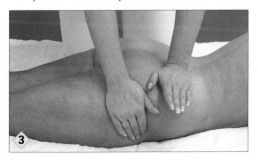

4 Glide your thumbs firmly up and over the buttocks in a line from the top of the leg up towards the

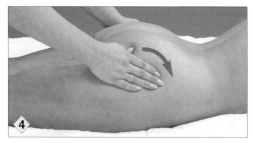

lower back. Do this four times, following an
imaginary line further towards the outside of the
buttock each time, and then go over each of these
lines again.

5 Place one hand on top of the other and point them
   both, keeping your fingers relaxed but straight.

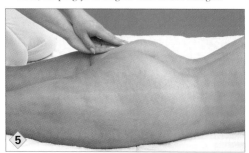

Press your fingers into the muscle of the buttocks and work the muscle deeply by rotating the fingers, building up pressure gradually, and decreasing it after about ten seconds. Work all over both buttocks.

6 Finish working on the buttocks by effleuraging slowly again, as in step 1. Gradually decrease the pressure over about a minute until your touch is hardly detectable. Cover the buttocks with a towel.

7 Keeping one hand on your partner, move to stand at their feet. Cover one leg with a towel and work on the other. Now effleurage the back of the leg from just above the ankle to the top of the thigh. Use your body weight to apply firm pressure, but release the pressure so it is very light over the back of the knee. Reapply it above the knee.

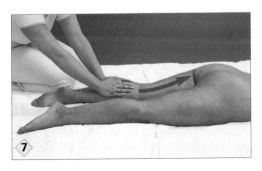

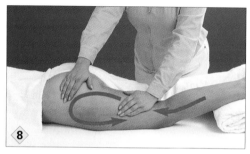

8 When you reach the top, sweep your hands round the outer thigh to return to the starting position. Make sure your inside hand does not move too far up the inside thigh as this may feel invasive to your partner. Repeat the effleurage twice.

9 Use alternate hands to effleurage firmly from the heel to the back of the knee. Move each hand around the calf away from the centre as you move it up towards the knee. Repeat this five times.

10 Use deeper pressure now, by placing your hands around the calf just above the ankle. Lean your body weight into the stroke as you push up the calf, stopping short of the back of the knee. Bring your hands lightly back down the sides of the calf, and repeat five times.

11 Move to stand beside the leg you are working on. Wrap your hands around the calf in opposite

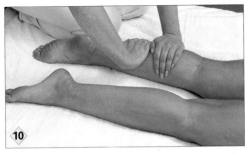

directions, holding the muscles between the thumb and fingers. Now pull one hand towards you as you push the other away from you. Do not merely move the skin (which would be painful) but make sure you are lifting and twisting the underlying muscle. Do this all over the calf for about a minute.

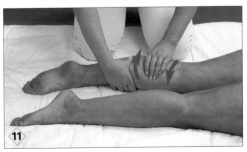

12 Return to your partner's feet, and place your outside hand around the calf so that your thumb rests flat across the centre of the back of it, just above the ankle. Push your thumb firmly up the back of the calf, increasing the pressure as you go, and stopping short of the back of the knee. As you finish the movement, begin it again at the ankle with the other hand. Repeat this twice.

13 Stand beside your partner and effleurage the back of the thigh by placing the heels of your hands either side of the thigh just above the back of the knee, with the hands facing out. Stroke firmly up the leg to the base of the buttock. Return your hands more lightly to the starting position, and repeat twice.

14 Cup your hands around the bottom of the thigh, facing inwards. Lean your weight into your hands

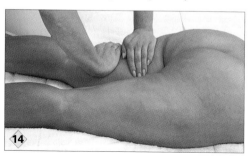

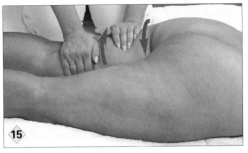

15

and push firmly and deeply up the back of the thigh. Return your hands down the sides of the thigh and repeat twice.

15 Place both your hands alongside each other at the base of the thigh. Grip the muscle in each of your cupped hands, and push away from you with one hand as you pull towards you with the other. You should be lifting, squeezing and wringing the muscle. Work your way right up the thigh.

16 Effleurage the whole leg again, from the ankle to the top of the thigh, easing the pressure over the back of the knee. Do this five times, then a further five times during which you gradually lighten the pressure until only your fingertips are touching the skin. Cover the leg with a towel and repeat the whole back of the leg massage on the other leg.

17 Ask your partner to turn over, and make them comfortable on their back. Take the pillow that was under the feet and replace it under the knees. Cover the leg you have just worked on with a towel, and uncover the other leg. Effleurage the front of the leg for about half a minute, working from the ankle to the top of the thigh.

18 Flex the knee and place the foot flat. Push the heel of your hand around the outside of the lower leg, working your way up to the knee and back down to the ankle. Repeat this effleurage twice. Lay the leg back down.

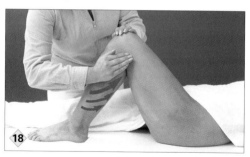

19 Place both hands just above the knee, heels of the hands together and your fingers wrapped around the leg. Using your body weight to exert pressure, push the heels of your hands down towards your

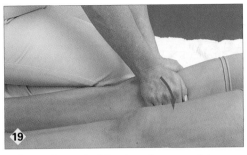

fingers. Return both hands to the centre of the thigh and repeat, working up the leg. Then work up the leg with each hand in turn.

20 Place your hands flat across the front of the thigh, and knead the muscle back and forth from hand to hand five times. Effleurage the thigh and then repeat the kneading.

21 Now pummel the outer thigh, keeping your hands in contact with the skin to avoid percussing. Work up and down the outside of the thigh five times. Effleurage the area afterwards by stroking lightly three or four times.

22 To work on the knee, hold it underneath with the fingers of both hands, leaving your thumbs free to work on the joint. Put both thumbs together at the top of the knee, in the groove around the outside of

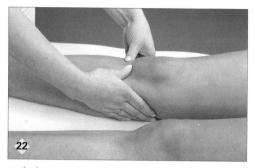

the kneecap. Press firmly but not too deeply into each natural indentation as you work round the kneecap to the bottom of it.

23 Effleurage the whole front of the leg, from the ankle to the top of the thigh, for about 30 seconds. The strokes should become increasingly lighter until they are barely perceptible. Cover the leg with a towel and repeat the treatment on the other leg.

FEET

A foot massage is very relaxing, and can benefit the whole body whether or not you are following reflexology techniques. There are numerous nerve endings in the feet, and stimulating these is a tonic for the rest of the system.

GETTING READY

- Put a pillow under the foot you are working on.

- If you are giving a foot massage alone, your partner can sit in a comfortable chair with their feet up; possibly with the foot you are working on in your lap.

- Many people have ticklish feet. If you encounter this problem, use firm strokes and apply a little more pressure. If this doesn't work, it may be better to avoid the ticklish areas or, if they are widespread, leave the foot massage until another day.

1 Begin by holding the foot between the palms of your hands, and stroking firmly along the foot towards the toes. Glide back and repeat this effleurage five times.

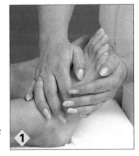

2 Place one hand flat against the sole of the foot, so that the heel

of your hand fits into the instep. Use your other hand to hold the ankle. Lean in to your hand so that it pushes slowly into the foot towards the knee. Hold the foot stretched in this position for ten seconds and release the pressure. Repeat.

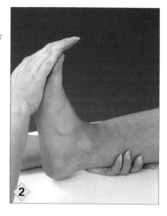

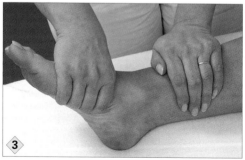

3 You are now going to stretch the foot in the opposite direction. Put one hand on top of the ankle, and wrap the other around the top of the foot. Lean into your hand to stretch the foot downwards slowly. Ask your partner to tell you when you have reached the point where it is about to become uncomfortable, and stop there. Hold the stretch for ten seconds and then release. Repeat.

4 Starting near the toes, wrap your hands around the foot so that the heels of your hands meet in the middle. Push them firmly apart, so that the heel of each hand moves towards the fingers. Repeat, working along the foot towards the ankle.

5 Hold the heel with one hand, and wrap the fingers of the other hand around the top of the foot,

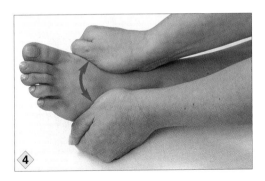

leaving the thumb free to work on the sole. Press the thumb into the sole of the foot and work it round in a small circle. Repeat this movement all over the base of the foot.

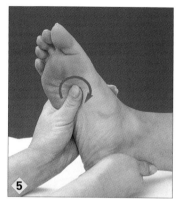

6 Now wrap the fingers of both hands around the top of the foot so that the thumbs meet on the sole of the foot, just below the toes. Push your thumbs firmly apart towards the edges of the foot. Work along, repeating this movement over the whole of the sole of the foot.

7 Hold the ankle with one hand, and with the other hold the big toe between the thumb and forefinger. Hold the sides of the toe, not the top and bottom, and hold near the base. Squeeze firmly and pull the toe gently as you slide your thumb and finger up and off the end of it. Repeat with each toe in turn.

8 Effleurage the whole foot again by sandwiching the foot between your hands and stroking firmly along the foot towards the toes. Repeat this five times. Now repeat the foot massage on the other foot.

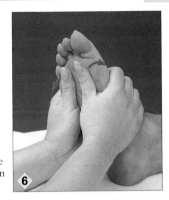

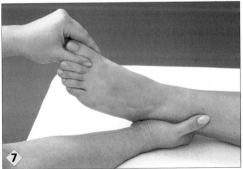

ARMS

Many of the nerves in the skin of the arms are related
to the chest organs, so an arm massage is beneficial
for the chest as well. This makes it especially useful if
you are massaging someone who is not fit enough for
a whole body massage. If you are giving someone an
arm massage alone, you can adapt this massage so that
your partner is sitting rather than lying down.

1 Lift the shoulder with both hands so that one hand
   slips beneath the shoulder blade. The tips of your
   fingers should just reach the spine. Place your other
   hand flat on the chest, fingers towards the shoulder,
   with the heel of the hand in the groove between
   your partner's chest and shoulder.

GETTING READY

- Have your partner lie on their back with a small
  pillow or folded towel under their head. Place
  another small pillow under the arm you are
  working on.

- Cover the body and upper legs with a towel,
  leaving the arms uncovered.

- Don't massage over any recent fractures,
  inflamed joints, or recent scars.

- Avoid heavy pressure on the funny bone, at the
  front of the elbow joint.

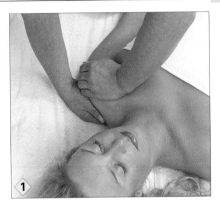

2 Hold this position for a few seconds, and then squeeze your hands together and pull them both slowly off the edge of the shoulder.

3 Hold your partner's hand level with your chest, and with your other hand effleurage the arm from wrist to shoulder. Stroke firmly up the arm and then return down the inside of the arm more lightly. Repeat five times. (*See illustration 3 on p. 80.*)

4 Lay the upper arm on the pillow, and rest the hand against your stomach. Effleurage the forearm only by circling it with your hand, your thumb on the inside of the wrist, and stroking firmly from wrist to elbow. Repeat five times, using alternate hands.

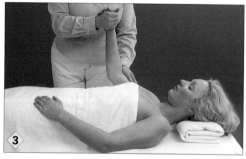

5 Now apply petrissage to the same area. Squeeze up and down the forearm with both hands close together, and squeezing alternately. Do this for about 30 seconds.

6 Place both hands around the wrist so that the thumbs meet in the centre of the inside of the wrist.

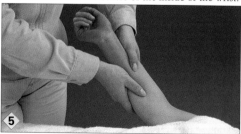

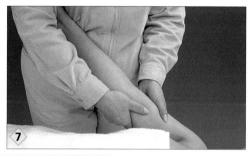

Apply deep effleurage from wrist to elbow. Repeat five times.

7 Raise the upper arm and, keeping the whole arm straight, keep it in place by holding the hand and forearm between your chest and your upper arm. You can now work on the top half of the arm. Effleurage the upper arm from elbow to shoulder. Repeat five times.

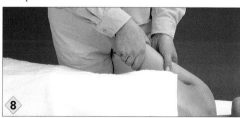

8 Squeezing back and forth from hand to hand, knead the upper arm for about 20 seconds working up to the shoulder and back down. Then effleurage five times. (*See illustration 8 on p. 81.*)

9 Lift the whole arm so that the wrist is directly above the shoulder. Effleurage firmly from wrist to shoulder with one hand, while holding your partner's hand in your other hand. Repeat twice, then change hands and effleurage three more times. Lay the arm back down by your partner's side, and repeat the massage on the other arm.

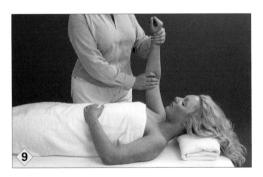

HANDS

Just as the nerves in the arm are related to those in the chest, so the nerves in the hand are related to those in

GETTING READY

- Work on the hands as a continuation of the arm massage, with your partner still lying on their back, towels over the body down to the knee.

- Rest your partner's elbow on a small pillow, with the elbow bent.

- You might prefer to use a hand cream instead of oil for this part of the massage.

- Avoid working over any areas which have been recently injured or which are swollen or inflamed.

the neck. So a hand massage eases pressure at the neck as well as relaxing the hand itself. A hand massage can easily be given on its own to someone who is sitting comfortably in a chair, as well as being given as part of a complete body massage.

1 Begin by simply holding your partner's hand sandwiched between your own for a few moments.

2 Effleurage the hand by sliding both hands lightly towards the forearm and back to the fingertips. Repeat this five times. (*See illustration 2 on p. 84.*)

3 Wrap your hands around your partner's hand so

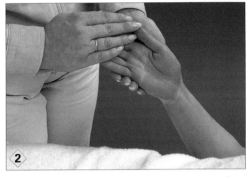

that the heels of your hands meet on the back of it. Lean into the heels of your hands as you push them apart, towards the edge of the hand, without sliding your fingers. Return to the starting position and repeat twice.

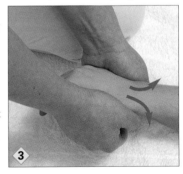

4 Hold the hand palm down with your fingers underneath it, leaving your thumbs free to massage the back of the hand. Using both thumbs, squeeze all over the bones and the grooves between them for about 30 seconds.

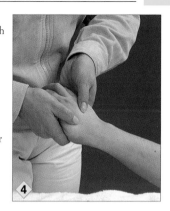

5 Return to the same starting position, but this time effleurage the back of the hand with your thumbs flat. Press lightly and move your thumbs apart as you stroke from the knuckles outwards.

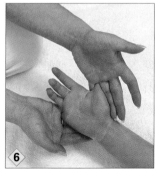

Work down the hand in this way to the wrist.

6 Sandwich your partner's thumb between the little and ring fingers of one hand, and their little finger between your other little and ring fingers. Stretch the palm slightly, and support the hand from underneath with your fingers.

7 Now rotate your thumbs in small circles all over the palm, applying light but firm pressure.

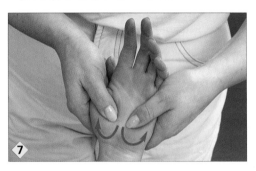

8 Turn the hand over again, palm down. Support it underneath with one hand. With the thumb and forefinger of the other hand, squeeze the base of the little finger and slide your thumb and finger up it. Give the finger a final squeeze as you pull your fingers off the end of it. Repeat with the other fingers and, finally, the thumb.

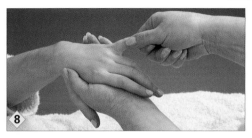

9 Support your partner's forearm with one hand. Put the back of your other hand under the forearm and slide it up under the hand.

10 Pull your hand up so that you can interlace your fingers between your partner's fingers. Holding them firmly, bend your own fingers upwards and

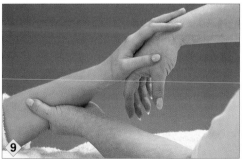

back towards yourself. Repeat twice.

11 Support your partner's hand in one of your own and, with the other, tap lightly with your fingertips together all over the front and back of the hand for about 20 seconds.

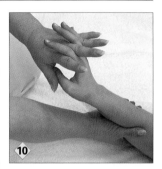

12 Complete the hand massage by effleuraging the whole hand between your own hands for about half a minute. The strokes should become increasingly

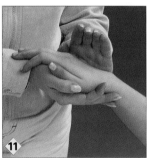

light, until only your fingertips are touching the skin; make sure you are still supporting the hand, however. Lay the hand down on the stomach and repeat the massage on the other hand.

ABDOMEN

The muscles of the abdomen are important, and often overlooked in massage. However, abdominal massage is hugely beneficial, and can help with conditions such as constipation and bloatedness. This part of the body can be ticklish; if this becomes a problem, return to firm effleurage strokes.

GETTING READY

- Your partner should be lying on their back, with a towel over the chest and shoulders, and another from the hips to the knees.

- Avoid massaging over recent scar tissue.

- Do not massage if there are any inflamed organs (for example, appendicitis, colitis).

- Do not massage for an hour after a large meal.

- Do not use heavy pressure during pregnancy, or during the first few days of menstruation.

- It is better if your partner does not talk during an abdominal massage, since it becomes hard to give the massage if the muscles are tightened.

- Avoid massaging the abdomen when your partner has a full bladder.

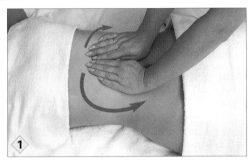

1 Lightly effleurage the abdomen starting with your
  hands flat just above the navel, beside each other.
  Glide your hands apart, round and down either
  side of the abdomen, then back in and up the
  middle to the starting position. Repeat five times.

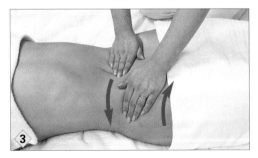

2 Place one hand on top of the other and effleurage the abdomen clockwise ten times.

3 Place your hands on opposite sides of the bottom of the abdomen, fingers pointing away from you and hands flat. Your far hand should be hooked over the side of the body. Push the hand nearest you away as you bring the far hand back towards you, so that they change positions. This should be a slow, strong movement but do not lean too heavily on the abdomen. Repeat, working up to the base of the ribs.

4 Knead the abdomen by picking up flesh between the thumb and fingers of one hand, without pinching, and pushing it towards the other hand. This hand should take the flesh and push it back, setting up a slow, alternating rhythm between the hands. Knead along the far side of the abdomen, then along the centre, and finally work along the side nearest to you.

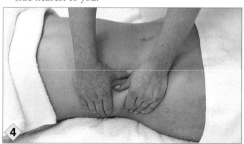

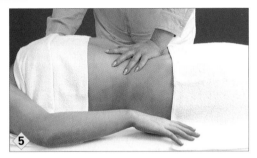

5 Place one hand in the centre of the abdomen, heel towards you and fingers outstretched. Do fanning, rotating the elbow and allowing the hand and fingers to follow the heel of the hand, giving slight friction and stretching. Rotate as far as you can and back again. Repeat twice.

6 Complete the abdominal massage by effleuraging once again starting with both hands flat just above the navel. Sweep your hands round down the sides, into the centre and back up again. Repeat five times, getting gradually lighter until only your fingertips are touching the skin. Cover the abdomen with a towel.

CHEST

The chest contains muscles which affect the ribcage,

GETTING READY

- Your partner should lie on their back with their arms by their sides and a small pillow or folded towel under their head.

- Cover your partner with a towel from the chest down.

- Don't apply heavy pressure anywhere on the chest.

- Don't massage over lumps, which should be checked by a doctor.

- Avoid massaging over any areas which have recently been scarred or fractured.

shoulder and upper arm. The sensitive tissue of a woman's breast means that you cannot massage the pectoral muscles, and many men find massage in this area uncomfortable, too. Relaxing the muscles of the chest helps prevent constricted breathing.

1 Stand behind your partner's head and place your hands at the top of the chest, fingers flat and facing each other, with the fingertips touching. Effleurage slowly and firmly, but without heavy pressure, by stroking your hands out to the shoulders. When you reach the shoulders, rotate the heels of your hands so that you scoop the fingers under the shoulders. (*See illustration 1 on p. 94.*)

2 Now bring the hands back along the top of the shoulders towards the neck, and let your fingers meet behind the neck.

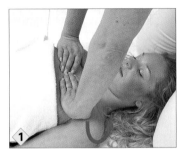

3 Cup one hand on top of the other, keeping the thumbs alongside the fingers, not on the throat. Bring your hands

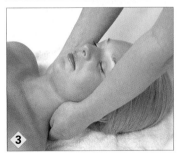

slowly towards you so that the neck is gently stretched. Release the hold and remove your hands by sliding them up round the back of the head. Return the hands to the top of the chest and repeat these three steps twice more.

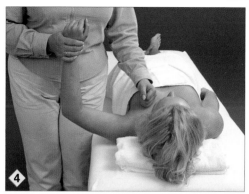

4 Move round to stand beside your partner. Hold
their arm at the wrist and pull it gently away from
the body so that the upper arm is raised a little.
Make your other hand into a soft fist and place it
on the area where the muscles of the chest, arm and
shoulder meet. Make circular pressing movements
with your fist around this area for about 20
seconds.

5 Now place the heel of your hand at the front of the
shoulder, with your fingers curled around the top of
it. Ask your partner to breathe in deeply and then
out. On the out breath, press the shoulder down
firmly for about five seconds, and shake the elbow
gently back and forth at the same time. Repeat the

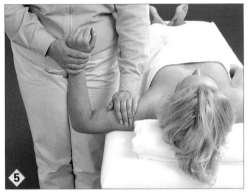

last two movements twice. (*See illustration above.*)

6 Still holding your partner's wrist, effleurage the arm from the wrist right through to the shoulder and on to the breastbone. Use a lighter stroke to return up the arm. Repeat five times. Now move around to the other side of your partner and repeat the last three steps on the other arm.

NECK

Stress and tension often collect in the neck, and are a common cause of headaches. Neck tension can build up over a long period of time, but massage is an excellent and deeply relaxing way to relieve it.

GETTING READY

- Have your partner lie on their back with a small pillow or a folded towel under their head. Cover them with a towel.

- You can adapt a neck massage so that your partner is sitting in a comfortable chair instead of lying down.

- Do not apply pressure directly to the spine.

1 Stand behind your partner's head, and effleurage lightly from the shoulders to the neck and face for about 15 seconds.

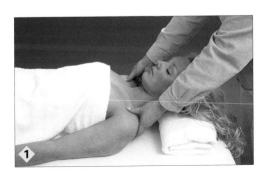

2 Without lifting it, roll the head gently from side to side twice, then roll it further to one side to let it rest.

3 Use one hand to steady the forehead, and with the other hand apply petrissage from

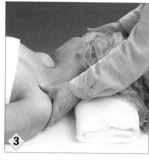

the shoulder to the back of the head and back out to the shoulder again. Squeeze gently, but do not squeeze the neck with your thumb. Repeat three times, then petrissage one way, from neck to shoulder, three more times.

4 Using both hands, lift the head clear of the pillow and rotate it to the other side without tilting or stretching it. Repeat the petrissage on this side.

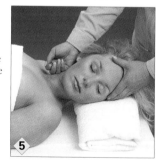

5 Curl your fingers and stroke the back of them gently up and down the muscle for about 20 seconds. This is the rotation muscle, which runs from just behind the ear to the centre of the chest. Lift the head in the same way as before and turn it back to face the other way. Repeat the stroking on the other side.

6 Finish by effleuraging both sides from the shoulders to the neck and face for about 15 seconds. Then effleurage more lightly from the shoulders to the neck and face and then up to the forehead lightly six times.

FACE

A face massage is an excellent treatment for headaches, whatever their cause. It also improves the circulation

GETTING READY

- Your partner can either lie with a small pillow or folded towel under the head, or sit in a chair.
- Ask your partner to remove any contact lenses so that you can massage over the eyes.
- Avoid massaging over infectious conditions such as spots.
- Don't use heavy pressure on the face.
- Check with your partner what depth of pressure feels comfortable for these movements.

to the face and revives the complexion. Some people swear by regular facial massage as an alternative to face-lifts, since it seems to take years off the face.

1 Stand behind your partner and rest your hands firmly on the forehead. Place your thumbs alongside each other in the centre of the forehead, with your fingers around the side of the head. Push your thumbs outwards across the forehead to the ears, making sure the pressure is even right along the thumbs.

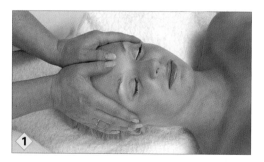

2 Bring the thumbs back to the centre and repeat the movement a little further up the forehead, following through the movement to the ears again. Keep repeating it up to the hairline.

3 Now place the thumbs back in the same position

but this time directly on the eyebrows. Draw the thumbs across the eyebrows and down to the ears. Repeat twice, finishing with the thumbs resting on the temples.

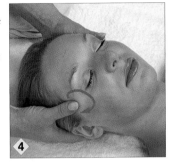

4 With your thumbs on the temples, press firmly and make small, clockwise circles very slowly for about 20 seconds.

5 Place your thumbs on the inside corners of the eyes

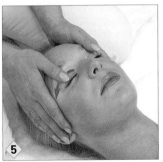

(make sure they are closed first). Draw your thumbs across the eyes with no pressure – so gently that you don't even drag the skin – and continue the stroke down to the ears. Repeat.

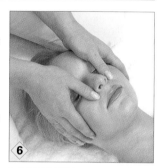

6 Move your thumbs to position them either side of the top of the nose. Slide them slowly down the nose to the outside corners of the nostrils. Do not use too much pressure or you will block the nostrils. Repeat twice. The final time you do this, keep your thumbs in the finish position and build up the pressure gradually, holding it for about ten seconds before releasing.

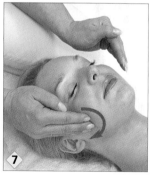

7 Place the pads of your three middle fingers on the part of the cheekbones nearest to the nose. Using slight pressure, circle the fingers slowly half a dozen times. Move the fingers to the centre of the cheekbones and repeat, and then to the outside edge of the cheekbones and repeat again.

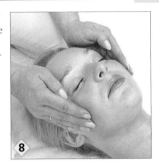

8 Move your three middle fingers down slightly so that they are next to the ears and just under the cheekbones. They should be on top of the jaw socket. Pressing slightly, rotate your fingers slowly three times.

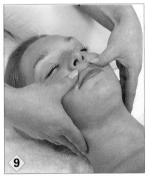

9 Place your fingers round behind your partner's neck, and bring your thumbs together to meet between the top lip and the nose. Pressing lightly, slide them out just beyond the edge of the top lip. Repeat twice.

10 Now reposition the thumbs to meet between the bottom lip and the chin. You can use a little more pressure here, and slide them outwards just beyond the edge of the bottom lip.

11 Hold the jaw either side of the chin between your thumb and fingers, making sure you don't touch the throat. Squeeze your fingers and thumbs together, and make small circles with your thumbs. Work your way like this along the bottom jaw to the ears.

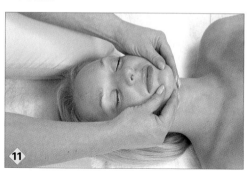

12 Continue this movement onto the ears, squeezing the lobe between fingers and thumb, and making small circles with your thumb up the outside of the ear.

13 Wrap your fingers around the ears so the heels of your hands are on top of the ears. Slowly draw your hands down without pulling the ears uncomfortably, until your hands slide off the ears. Repeat.

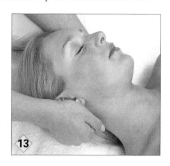

14 Effleurage the face from chin to temples five times, starting with one hand first, and beginning the movement with the second hand as you complete it with the first.

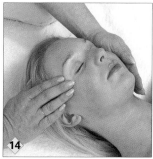

15 Drum the fingertips lightly all over the face except for the eyes and the tip of the nose. This is the tapping percussion stroke known as tapotement.

16 Effleurage the face again from chin to temples five times, and from forehead to temples five times. Finally, effleurage from chin to temples five more times, getting lighter each time until only the fingertips are touching the skin.

HEAD

A head massage is a wonderfully relaxing way to complete a full body massage, although you can give the head massage alone, which takes about five minutes, or add it to the end of a facial massage.

GETTING READY

- Have your partner lie on their back with their head resting on a small pillow or folded towel.

- Check whether your partner minds oil in their hair; if they do, wash your hands thoroughly if you have just been using it on any other part of the body.

- Check with your partner what depth of pressure feels comfortable for these movements.

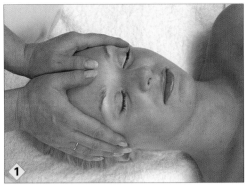

1 Place your thumbs alongside each other in the centre of the forehead, with your fingers around the side of the head. Press firmly with the whole thumb as you pull your thumbs back until the tips are level with the hairline.

2 Place one thumb over the other and apply pressure to the head for about five seconds. Release. Move the thumbs further back down the head and repeat. Keep repeating this movement as far back down the head as you can reach with your thumbs.

3 Return your thumbs to either side of the starting position on the hairline. Again, apply pressure for about five seconds and then release. Work back down the head again as far as you can.

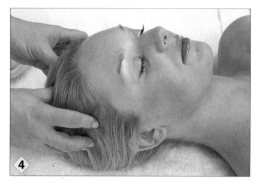

4 Place the finger pads on the head inside the
  hairline, roughly parallel with the line of the
  eyebrows. Apply pressure and rotate your fingers
  vigorously as if shampooing the hair. Work all over
  the head, including the base of the skull.

5 With your palms facing towards you, and the back
  of your hands against your partner's head, draw the
  fingers of each hand alternately through your
  partner's hair. Keep this movement flowing as you
  work over the entire head.

6 Rest one hand slowly on the head, fingertips on the
  hairline, with the other hand on top of it. Slowly
  press down until you have reached a firm but
  comfortable pressure. Maintain this for about ten

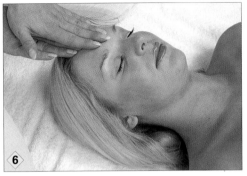

seconds, and then release the pressure so slowly
that your partner is barely aware of it. Remove the
top hand gradually, and then the lower hand.

SELF MASSAGE

BENEFITS

Although many massage strokes are impossible to use on yourself, and others are very uncomfortable, there are still many effective strokes which you can use or adapt to massage yourself.

You can use a full self massage treatment regularly – perhaps once a week – to relax you and help prevent many tension-related problems. You can also use self massage to treat many common problems, from period cramps to insomnia.

What's more, using massage strokes on yourself is a very good way to practise them so that you know how they feel to someone else when you treat them.

Self massage is deeply relaxing, and can help to ease tensions throughout the day. In parts of China, workers regularly massage themselves as part of their daily routine.

It is also an excellent way of giving massage to very tender parts of the body; it can be hard to relax and allow anyone else to give a massage if you are worried the pressure might be too painful. But you can always trust yourself to massage a damaged joint, or a tender abdomen.

GETTING READY

- Choose a quiet, private area, just as you would if you were giving a massage to someone else.
- Make sure you are warm enough.
- Sit on a comfortable upright chair or on the floor, or lie down.
- If you don't have time for a full self massage, don't rush the sequence. It is better to do part of it only – whichever part you feel you want or need to do.
- You will probably find it easier to use oil, although you can omit this for the face and head. If you are giving yourself an impromptu massage, perhaps to ease a particular pain, you can always manage without oil if you don't have any, but try to use it if you can.

FACE

1 Begin by closing your eyes and stroking your face with the flat of your hands. Stroke from the centre of the forehead out to the temples three times, from the centre of the nose out over the cheekbones three times, and from the centre of the mouth out along the jawline three times.

2 Using the pads of your three middle fingers, circle all over the face pressing firmly, and feeling for any areas of tension. (*See illustration 2 on p. 112.*)

3 Using your thumbs and forefingers, gently squeeze the earlobes and pull them. Work all around the edges of the ears squeezing and pulling.

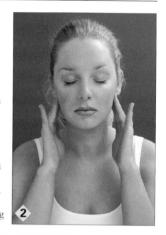

4 Now place your hands flat over your ears, so you can hear the sound of the sea. This is very relaxing. Pressing gently on the ears, ease them back, down, round and up in a circle. Repeat.

5 Tap very lightly with the pads of your fingers under your eyes and over the eyelids.

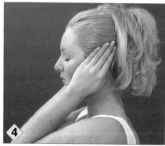

HEAD

1 Place the palms of your hands on your temples, and rest your fingers on top of your head. Using firm pressure, make slow, circling movements with the heels of your hands. Work all over the front and 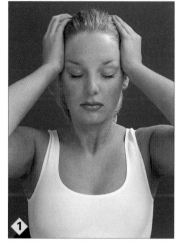 sides of the head, and as much of the back as you can reach comfortably.

2 Run your hands through your hair, one after the other, so that you pull gently on the roots of the hair. Work at an easy pace all over the scalp.

3 Using both hands alternately, pluck all over the scalp in a percussion movement to help stimulate the circulation and to wake yourself up.

SELF MASSAGE FOR THE CIRCULATION

1 Fold a bath towel lengthwise and hold the ends in
  your hands with the towel around your shoulders.
  Pull the towel back and forth across your shoulders
  to create a warming friction. Work the towel up to
  your neck and down your back for about a minute.
  Rest and repeat twice.

2 Now move the towel to your lower back, still
  holding the ends with your hands and passing the
  towel back and forth under your arms. Again create
  a warm friction for about a minute, then rest and
  repeat twice.

NECK AND SHOULDERS

1 Place the fingers of
  both hands at the
  top of the neck
  behind the ears.
  Bend your head
  slightly forwards to
  stretch the neck
  muscles a little.
  Now use the pads
  of your fingers to
  make circling
  movements either
  side of the spine
  (but not directly on
  it). Work slowly

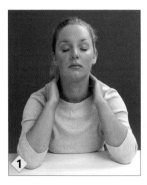

down the neck.
Repeat twice.

2 Bring your right hand up to your left shoulder near the neck, and lean your head a little away from it. Squeeze the shoulder muscle deeply between the heel of your hand and the fingers. Slowly rotate the shoulder

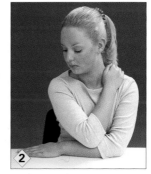

twice. Now work your way along the top of the shoulder, squeezing the muscle, from the neck to the shoulder joint. Repeat twice.

3 Starting nearest the neck, place the pads of your fingers on the shoulder muscle, and make circling movements deep into the muscle. Work along to the shoulder joint and repeat twice.

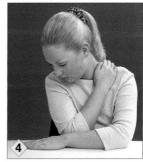

4 Support your right elbow on a table top or with the
left hand. Make a loose fist with your right hand
and pummel your left shoulder with it by bouncing
it up and down on the muscle. Begin gently and
increase the pressure gradually. Work out along the
shoulder from the neck to the shoulder joint. Do
not raise your fist far from your neck and shoulder.
Continue for about 20 seconds. Now repeat the last
three steps on the other shoulder.

ARMS

1 Effleurage your arm
from the wrist up to the
shoulder, then round the
shoulder joint and, more
lightly, back down again.
Repeat three times.

2 Squeeze the muscle at
the top of your outer
arm between the heel of
your hand and the
fingers. Work down to
the elbow, squeezing the
muscle. Return to the
top of the arm and
squeeze down the inside
of the upper arm.

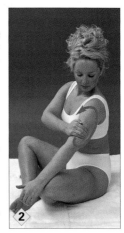

3 Press your knuckles into
the muscle inside your

upper arm and make circling movements with the knuckles, all over the upper arm and then the lower arm.

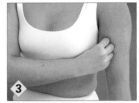

4 Wrap your fingers around your elbow and rotate in a large circle right around the elbow joint. Then use small circles to work your fingers into the grooves all over the elbow joint, massaging it thoroughly.

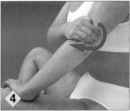

5 Working with your forearm instead of your hand, roll it down the forearm you are working on from the elbow to the wrist. Repeat twice. Repeat the whole sequence for the arms on the other side.

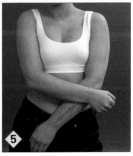

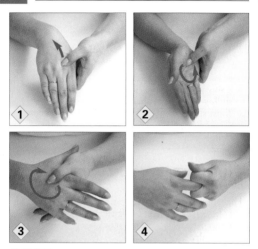

HANDS

1 Begin by rubbing the palms of your hands together to warm them up. Then take one hand in the fingers of the other, and use the thumb to stroke down the back of the hand between the tendons, from the knuckles to the wrist. Apply firm, deep pressure.

2 Now work on the palm. Press your thumb firmly into the base of the palm and stroke it down and out to the edge in a fanning motion. Repeat four

times. Then make small circles with your thumb all over the palm of the hand, pressing firmly.

3 Work on the back of the hand with the thumb. Press it firmly down and make small circles all over the back of the hand.

4 Using your knuckles, pull on the little finger, sliding up from the base of the finger to the tip. Twist slightly as you pull up and off the end of the finger. Repeat with the other fingers and the thumb. Repeat the whole sequence on the other hand.

HYDROTHERAPY SELF MASSAGE FOR INSOMNIA

1 Get out of bed and hold each wrist under running cold water for about a minute to cool it (but not freeze it). Dab the water off with a towel, but don't rub it dry. Go back to bed and lie on your side with your hands tucked under your crossed arms.

2 Close your eyes and breathe deeply as if you were already asleep. As your hands become warmer, the blood flow to your brain will reduce, helping you to fall asleep.

CHEST

1 Wrap your fingers under your armpit and squeeze the pectoral muscle between your fingers and the heel of your hand. Work thoroughly into the muscle

for about 20 to 30 seconds, then change to work on the other side of your chest.

2 Place the palms of your hands with fingertips touching in the centre of your upper chest. The fingers should be splayed out. Stroke outwards, with your fingertips running between your ribs, using deep pressure. Continue the movement to the edges of the ribcage, then return to the starting position and repeat.

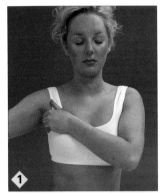

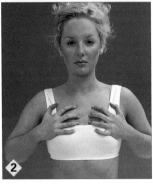

ABDOMEN

1 Place one hand flat on the abdomen and stroke in a circular movement, running clockwise (the direction of the intestinal tract). The stroke should start small, and enlarge to encompass the whole abdomen, from the ribcage to the pubic bone. Then bring the circles back down in size again. Apply as much pressure as is comfortable.

2 Using both hands, pick up the flesh on your abdomen and squeeze it between your fingers and thumbs. Roll the flesh to knead it, using as much pressure as is comfortable. Work over the entire abdomen like this. It can help to lie on your back, and bend your knees to the right as you work on the left side, and to the left as you work on the right side.

3 Place the fingers of one hand on top of the other, apply static pressures all over the abdomen, holding each for about five seconds. Follow the clockwise circular movement around the abdomen that you made earlier.

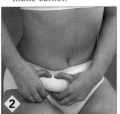

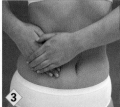

SELF MASSAGE FOR CONSTIPATION

1 Make a fist with your right hand and gently press it around the edge of the abdomen in a clockwise direction. Increase the pressure, and focus on pressing most deeply as you push your fist down the left side of your abdomen.

LOWER BACK

1 Sit in an upright chair, or on the floor with your feet together and your knees flopped out to the side. Place the palms of both hands either side of the spine on the lower back and rub vigorously all over to warm the area and relieve tension.

2 Make your hands into fists and press them, thumb side towards your back, into either side of the base of the spine. Stroke up and down firmly.

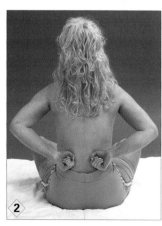

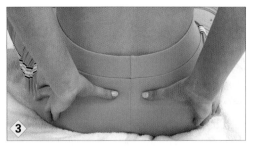

3 Press your thumbs either side of the lower spine and make firm, circling movements all around the area.

4 Finally, make loose fists and pummel all over the area, taking care to avoid the spine. Finish by effleuraging the area again with the palms of your hands.

LEGS

1 Sit on the floor or a firm sofa or bed with your legs out in front of you. Slightly raise the knee of the leg you are working on first. Effleurage the whole leg upwards from the ankle to the thigh, either using a hand over hand action, or with your hands either side of the leg stroking simultaneously – whichever is the most comfortable.

2 Squeeze the muscle at the top of your thigh between the fingers and the heel of one hand. Now

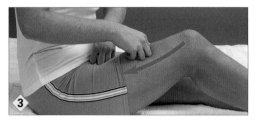

push it towards the other hand, and take it in the
fingers and heel of that hand. Knead the muscle by
pushing and squeezing from hand to hand
rhythmically. Work all over the top and back of the
thigh, and then on the calf muscles.

3 Press your knuckles into the muscle just above the
knee and slide your hands up the thigh, one after
the other. Work up the top of the thigh, then the
outside and then the inside.

4 Make loose fists and pummel the top and outside of
the thigh by bouncing your fists lightly on the
thigh. Focus on the upstroke as you pull your fist
up and away from the skin, but don't raise your
fists too high – keep them close to the body. Work
over the thigh for about 20 to 30 seconds.

5 With both hands, use the thumbs and the pads of
your middle fingers to work into the indentations of
the knee. Press gently but firmly and move your
fingers and thumbs in small circles all over the knee.

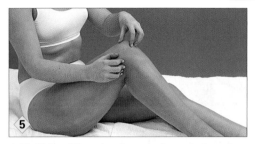

6 Finish by effleuraging the entire leg again from the ankle to the top of the thigh. Rest your leg back down and bend the other knee slightly. Repeat the whole sequence on the other leg.

FEET

1 Sit on a floor, bed or sofa with your legs out in front of you. Bend one knee outwards to rest the foot on the other knee. Hold the foot between the flats of your hands and rub them backwards and forwards to stroke and warm up the foot.

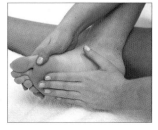

2 Place your foot down flat in front of you, and wrap your hands round the foot so that your fingers are underneath it and the heels of your hands meet in the middle of the top of your foot. Push the heels of your hands out across your foot as you push your fingers up into the sole, so that you stretch the top of your foot. Repeat five times.

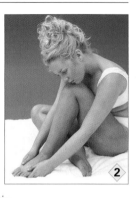

3 Leave your fingers where they are and use your thumbs on top of the foot to press in little circles all over the foot.

4 Now place the thumbs at the end of the outer tendons between the toes, and stroke firmly up the foot to the ankle along the furrow. Move the thumbs in to work on the other two tendons. Repeat.

5 Replace your foot on the opposite knee so you can work on the sole. Wrap your fingers around the top of the foot and place your thumbs in the centre of the ball of the foot. Work your thumbs in small circles all over the sole, including the heel.

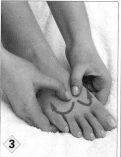

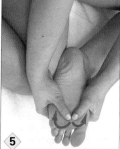

6 Hold your heel with one hand and use the other to extend and flex the toes to increase suppleness.

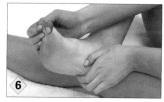

7 With a loose fist, pummel the sole of your foot with a light action, striking it loosely all over from toes to heel, including the sides of your foot. Continue for about 20 seconds.

8 In the same position, switch from a pummelling action to a hacking stroke. Keeping your hand close to the foot, strike it with the side of your hand so

that your hand bounces off. Remember to keep your hand and wrist relaxed.

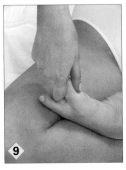

9 Hold each toe in turn between your thumb and forefinger. Squeeze gently and pull on the toe, twisting slightly, as you slide your finger and thumb right down the toe and off.

10 Complete the foot massage by returning to the first step and placing the flats of your hands on the top and bottom of your foot. Rub them gently backwards and forwards to relax the foot. Now repeat the entire sequence on the other foot.

QUICK SELF MASSAGE FOR THE FEET

1 Stand in cool water to a depth of about three or four inches. Lift the feet out of the water alternately. Now dry them and sit down on an upright chair. Place a tennis ball under one of your feet and roll your foot backwards and forwards along it for about a minute. Then change to the other foot.

MASSAGE WITH
SPECIAL SUBJECTS

During our lives our bodies undergo many changes such as the tremendous growth between birth and adulthood, pregnancy in women, the ageing process, stress, injury and illness.

Massage at these times can be very effective in relaxing us and allowing our bodies to undergo the changes with ease and efficiency. If we are tense and ill-prepared we will find change harder to adapt to and accept. If we are supple and relaxed we can be more adaptable and responsive.

In this chapter we will look at how massage can help us during pregnancy and also how massage can be very beneficial for babies and children.

We will look at some self help techniques as well as getting others to massage us.

Massage for Pregnancy

There is no greater change that can happen to a woman's body than pregnancy, during the forty weeks it takes from conception to birth. And the change is dramatic both physically and emotionally. For the woman's partner, using and giving massage is a wonderful way of both supporting her and feeling useful himself. It allows the man to care for his partner in a very real and practical way as well as providing comfort and help.

During pregnancy there is little in the way of medicines and drugs that a woman can take to relieve pain and discomfort and massage, if used correctly, is both safe and effective in these cases. The woman's body

BENEFITS OF MASSAGE IN PREGNANCY

- Stimulates lymphatic and circulatory systems
- Decreases back pain
- Lowers blood pressure
- Improves sleep
- Increases relaxation and lowers stress levels
- Helps minimise the incidence of varicose veins
- Prevents stretch marks
- Regulates bowel movements
- Relieves aches and cramps especially in the legs

undergoes such enormous changes in a very short space of time that all women will experience some discomfort and pain to a greater or lesser extent. Massage can help relieve pain as well as keeping her body supple and toned.

POSTURE DURING PREGNANCY

During pregnancy women gain around an extra 13 kilos on average as well as changing their overall body shape quite considerably. The common postural defect during pregnancy is to throw the abdomen forward to compensate for the extra weight being carried.

Unfortunately although this seems to alleviate the tension in the neck and shoulders, it has the effect of forcing the back to curve backwards increasing the likelihood of severe back strain with its corresponding back pain. Over 80% of women experience considerable back pain during pregnancy.

Although massage can do a lot to relieve the pain it is best to try to avoid it in the first place, by improving the posture and avoiding curving the back, as mentioned above. The woman should endeavour to maintain a straight back at all times. Weight distribution should be maintained evenly on both legs; high heels should be avoided; shoulders should be pulled back; the pelvis should be tipped up and back; the spine should be lengthened as much as possible and the crown of the head held high with the chin tucked in.

MASSAGE FOR THE ABDOMEN

Massaging the woman's abdomen can be a wonderful way for her partner to be in touch with the developing baby. This massage should be carried out with sooth-

RULES FOR MASSAGE IN PREGNANCY

- Except in the very early stages of pregnancy don't carry out any massage with the woman in the prone (face down) position.

- Only apply gentle, soft effleurage movements.

- Don't use deep pressure applications on the lower back or the abdomen.

- Don't use tapotement.

- Certain essential oils should not be used in pregnancy; see the charts in the aromatherapy section on pp. 182 and 183.

- Take extreme care, especially during the first trimester, of the abdomen and lower back. If in any doubt, avoid these areas.

- Don't use massage to try to treat any cases of sudden swelling in the ankles, feet, hands, wrists or face. These should be referred to your GP immediately.

ing, gentle strokes and has been found to calm very active babies – those that kick a lot – even in the womb. You can do this massage up to around twenty weeks with your partner lying on her back if she still feels comfortable enough to do so. After that get her to lie on her side and support her head with pillows and place another pillow between her legs for extra comfort.

1 Get your partner to lie on one side and kneel behind her. Gently stroke her abdomen by beginning in the middle with one hand and drawing it up over her stomach. As soon as one hand begins its stroke use your other hand to replace it, so a continuous stroking movement is effected. As one hand ends its movement by lightly stroking her lower back it begins again in the lower centre of her stomach.

2 Use both hands to stroke a large circle around her stomach with one hand following the other. Use a clockwise movement and, as one arm crosses the other, lift your hand off and begin again, making a full circle. This isn't a deep massage in any way but a light stroking, a soothing caress to provide warmth, closeness, comfort and tenderness.

3 Again using the same position just use one hand to begin a light, sweeping stroke in a wide circle around the abdomen. Gradually decrease the circle until you have spiralled into the navel. Here you can just use a tiny circle around the navel with a very light touch.

LOWER BACK AND LEGS MASSAGE

As it is very rare for a woman to find it comfortable to lie in the prone (face down) position during the later stages of pregnancy, you can massage her lower back and legs with her either kneeling or standing up taking most of her weight by leaning on a wall.

1 Get your partner to take her weight by leaning on a wall. You can kneel beside her. To ease any lower back pain hold her buttocks in your fingers and press deeply into the centre of each buttock with your thumbs. Hold the pressure for a few seconds and then release. Don't press tightly enough to cause pain but with sufficient pressure to sink your thumbs quite deeply, Make sure your finger nails are short and smooth.

2 For easing pain in the legs again get your partner to lean forwards and take her weight on the wall. Kneel beside her and gently effleurage down the back of her legs. Stroke gently but firmly, and allow your partner to shift her weight from one leg to the other as you massage each leg.

FOOT MASSAGE

Most women experience swollen ankles and feet at some stage during pregnancy and also suffer from aching feet. You can help by massaging these areas not only to alleviate the swellings and aches but also to revitalise her whole body.

Your partner will probably find it most comfortable to sit in a semi-reclined position with her feet propped up on a cushion on a low table. Or you could get her to lie across a sofa with her feet in your lap if you both find it comfortable.

1 Hold the top of your partner's foot between your hands and stroke both hands firmly down towards her ankles. Allow your hands to return to her toes without losing contact and again firmly run your hands, palms innermost, towards her ankles. Do this several times.

2 Once your partner is used to your touch on her foot cup your fingers around her heel. Use your other hand to support her ankle. The hand cupping her heel can now massage quite deeply using the thumb only to press into the area around her heel and into the sole.

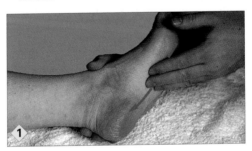

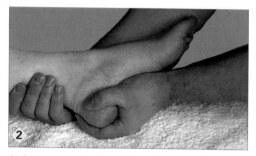

3 Again supporting her ankle with one hand use the other hand to massage with your finger tips the whole of the bottom of her foot. Use circular movements with increased pressure each time you bring your fingers down towards the ankle. Gradually make the circles larger until you reach the toes. Gently pull each toe outwards away from the ankle. Squeeze and release. Finish by again using both hands palm inwards to stroke along the foot towards the ankle. Then do the other foot.

BACK MASSAGE DURING PREGNANCY

In the later stages of pregnancy you won't be able to massage your partner with her in the prone (face down) position, but it is her back that will require the most attention. So get her to kneel and lean forwards onto a well padded support – perhaps a duvet folded several times or a large pile of cushions. Make sure her face and head are level with her back and not lower. You can begin this massage with her sitting upright as you attend to her shoulders and allow her to slowly move forwards as you massage her back.

1 To begin keep your left hand on her right shoulder to stabilise both of you, and use your right hand to lightly massage her right shoulder blade in a circular movement. As your hand reaches the top of her back change hands and massage her left shoulder blade and, as you do so, bring your right hand up to support you both on her left shoulder. Keep doing this until you work up a smooth and even rhythm and can feel warmth being generated beneath your hands.

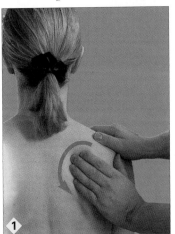

2 Begin by kneading the top of her right shoulder. Rhythmically squeeze and roll the flesh with alternate hands and use your thumbs to roll the flesh up from the shoulder blade towards your fingers. Don't squeeze too hard but be firm enough to 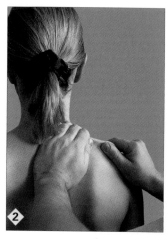 generate warmth. Feel for any knotted lumps of tension and work these out by increased rolling. Then do the same to her left shoulder.

3 You can use your right hand fingertips to massage the area around her shoulder blade. You may need to support the front of her body using your arm to prevent her toppling forward, as you will need to press quite hard. Apply deep circular movements along the edge of the shoulder blade and push up and under the bone. Finish off by stroking the

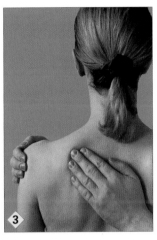

whole area with light strokes and then repeat the whole process with the area around her left shoulder blade.

4 Now get your partner slowly to take her weight on her arms by gently falling forwards onto her pile of cushions. Make sure her back is level and flat. Kneel behind her and place both hands on her lower back either side of her backbone. Push your hands up her back towards her shoulders. When you reach her shoulders squeeze them firmly and then stroke down each of her arms to her wrists.

5 Bring your hands back up her arms lightly and then stroke down the sides of her body, around the hips, down the legs to her ankles and then around her buttocks and back to your starting position. Repeat these two steps several times.

MASSAGE FOR BABIES

Probably the best skill any parent can learn is to feel comfortable touching, holding and physically bonding with their child. Once a parent is confident physically with a child they also become much more at ease with the emotional side of child rearing. Bringing up a baby is no easy task. As soon as you think you've got it licked they'll change all the rules; just when you have learnt not to get stressed with them crawling they'll learn to walk. And so it goes on. They are built to learn – and learn they will. Babies never stay still educationally but are always striving to attain the next learning curve, master the next set of skills, accomplish the next development stage. And because they are so restless within themselves they too get stressed and tense.

BABIES NEED MASSAGE TOO

Massaging for both parent and child is therapeutic, relaxing, bonding and essential. Because children grow at such a tremendous rate they too will experience physical stress that needs relieving. This is why massage is so important to babies. In the West we aren't as easy with massaging small children as they are in, say, China or India, where it is much more a part of parenting. But we can certainly learn and, once learnt, massage becomes natural and important – just as much as cuddling, hugging and caressing your child.

There are however a few important guidelines which may not apply to adults but certainly do to very small babies; these are listed opposite.

DOS AND DON'TS OF BABY MASSAGE

- Don't wake a small baby to massage it; wait until he or she is awake.

- Never massage a baby if it seems distressed for any reason.

- Don't massage any area around an immunisation site for about 48 hours. After that you can gently massage the area especially if there is a residual lump.

- Don't massage a baby if it is in any way off colour or feeling unwell.

- Don't massage just before or after a feed.

- Make sure both the room and the baby are suitably warm.

- Make sure your hands are clean and your nails are short.

- Lie the baby on its back on a safe surface with a towel or cotton sheet under it.

- Use only the very lightest of unscented oils such as grapeseed or sweet almond.

- Always test the oil on a tiny patch of the baby's skin to see if it is allergic to it first. Keep any oil you use well away from the baby's eyes.

- Make sure you too are comfortable and enjoying giving the massage – it is not a chore to be endured but a delight to be enjoyed.

MASSAGING YOUR BABY WILL:

- Enhance your relationship with your child.

- Provide physical and emotional contact.

- Engender confidence in your handling your baby.

- Calm and soothe your baby.

- Stimulate your baby's immature immune, circulatory and digestive systems.

- Encourage your baby to know and relate to you.

1 Begin by cupping the baby's head in your hands and looking at them so they know what's happening to them. Hold their head in one hand and gently stroke with your finger-tips from the top of the nose out towards the forehead in a semi-circle. Stroke down the ears, round the jaw and back up the face alongside the nose several times. Change hands and do the other side of their face.

2 Change hands again and very gently with your thumb stroke up and across the top of the head, making sure you use extreme care with the fontanel. All of this face and head massage should be done without oil.

3 Warm a little oil in your hands. Rub it into your

palms and begin massaging each of your baby's arms. Roll them gently between your hands and stroke them up and down. Stroke the hands and fingers, which you can then gently roll and pull individually. Hold the baby's hands and bring them together across the baby's chest. Then relax them out to the sides. Do this several times.

4 Place your hands on your baby's stomach and very gently circulate them outwards and up the chest. As your hands reach the chest you can bring them back down the baby's sides and back across the stomach. This should be a light, gentle movement carried out smoothly.

5 Bring your baby's knees up to their stomach and gently rotate their legs. Stretch the legs out and massage them in much the same way as you did the arms. You can pay particular attention to the soles of their feet as most babies seem to love having this area massaged.

6 Sit the baby on your lap. Support the front of their body with your hand and wrist across the front of their chest. Your other hand can then massage their back by making small circles up and down the spine on ether side of the spine (but not directly on it). Stroke the baby's back up and down lightly with your fingertips. As your hands will be oily make especially sure the baby is securely supported by your other hand at all times.

Massage for Children

It is only natural that as children grow up the amount of physical contact with their parents tails off. This can be detrimental to both child and adult alike. However, children, especially teenagers, simply recoil from too much physical contact and you can't force it. But offer them a massage – perhaps only their legs to begin with after they've been playing hockey or football – and they will gladly agree. You can then re-establish physical contact and be of use to them at the same time. Once physical contact is reintroduced like this they will be much more amenable to you massaging them at other times.

Children undergo quite considerable stress both physically and emotionally and derive as much benefit from being massaged as adults – it's just getting them to submit to it that's the problem. Of course there are children, especially if they have been brought up to have a considerable amount of physical contact right from birth, who won't object at all. If you have more than one child you can get all the children to massage each other. This can result in a reduction of sibling rivalry as they bond better, are more used to physical contact with each other, and are more relaxed anyway because of the massage.

There are benefits in other ways, too: research done in the US on problem children has shown that a daily

MASSAGING CHILDREN

- If a child doesn't want to be cuddled offer a massage as an alternative and you may get better results.

- Don't force a child to be massaged if they simply don't want to be.

- Encourage them to return the favour and get them to massage you as well – don't expect great results but at least you are getting physical contact of a sort. And you may be surprised by their expertise.

- Encourage them to be part of the process by allowing them to help you make up any essential oils – and let them choose which oils they prefer.

massage greatly reduced problem behaviour, improved their sleep patterns and resulted in better general co-operation than in a similar control group who were only shown relaxation videos.

Above are some tips for massaging children.

1 Begin by gently kneading the back of their neck and rolling the flesh either side of their shoulders between your thumb and forefinger.

2 Stroke your hands up and down the back of the

neck. Use your fingers to make deep circular pressure movements all around the neck area but not
on the spine.

3 Hold and squeeze the muscles either side of the
neck on the top of the shoulders. Feel for any knotted lumps of tension and work hardest at those.

4 With your fingers stroke firmly from the centre of
the back outwards applying deeper pressure at the
sides. When you reach the edges of the back return
to the centre and start again. Again, concentrate on
any tension spots you find.

5 Have them lie down on their back, and kneel at
their feet. Place the foot between your knees and
bend the child's knee. Place your hands at the top
of their thigh and run one down quite firmly to the
knee. As it reaches the knee run the other down
while the first hand returns to the top of the thigh.
Run it down while the second hand is being

You can get children to give each other a pummelling massage by using the sides of their
hands to gently pummel their sibling's back. This
makes for a lot of fun, is extremely relaxing and
makes a great noise as well. Make sure they
don't hit the spine but only the back on either
side of it.

returned. Move your hands around the thigh so that all of it is massaged.

6 With the knee still bent you can now do the same procedure to the leg from the knee down to the ankle. You can also put both hands around the ankle and firmly pull your hands up to the knee. Repeat with the other leg.

MASSAGE FOR COMMON AILMENTS

Many common conditions can be eased or relieved using massage. And as well as treating someone else for these ailments you may also be able to treat yourself.

An alphabetical list of common ailments follows, and a description of the treatment. All these treatments incorporate strokes and movements which are detailed elsewhere in the earlier sections of this book if they are not described here. Some of the more common complaints, such as headaches, also have their own separate entry in the second half of the chapter.

If you have some complaint such as a tension headache, you can no doubt diagnose it yourself. But if you are at all uncertain of the diagnosis, or if your symptoms persist, you should always see a doctor.

Never attempt to treat any serious disorders with massage – refer to your GP if you are in any doubt or if your symptoms have persisted for more than a few days.

Abdominal bloating Give an abdominal massage, with the focus on effleuraging in a clockwise direction – the direction of the colon.

See p. 158–160 for other abdominal complaints.

Aching feet A foot massage will ease this, and regular foot massage will help prevent it. You could precede the massage by soaking the feet in warm water, perhaps with a few drops of essential oil such as lavender or rosemary added to it.

Backache Effleurage to the aching area can help ease backache by improving the circulation of both blood and lymph, as well as by relaxing the muscles. This also warms the area. Effleurage will help with backache whatever the cause, whether it is ligament injury, PMS or the aftereffects of pregnancy. For a reflexology treatment, try massaging the insteps of both feet.

Cellulite The aim here is to improve circulation of both blood and lymph, and break down fatty deposits. So use long effleurage strokes to pep up the circulation, and work on the fatty tissues with petrissage and deep kneading on thighs and buttocks.

Chilblains These are the result of poor circulation. Foot massage will help stimulate the circulation and alleviate the symptoms. Regular massage will help to prevent chilblains recurring.

Constipation Give an abdominal massage, with the focus on effleuraging in a clockwise direction.

Cramp Deep effleurage and kneading will help to ease the muscle tension which causes cramp, and will lengthen the contracted muscle fibres.

See also p. 168-169.

Calf cramps can also be dealt with by stretching and releasing the muscle; see p. 169.

Eye strain
This can cause headaches and blurred vision. To relieve it, lean the heels of your hands into your eyes for about 20 seconds, then rotate them in the eye sock-ets making large circles for a further ten seconds.

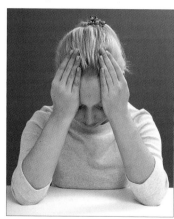

Foot problems See p. 170–172.

Fractured bones Do not massage during recovery, but massage can be very helpful to break up scar tissue later. Use deep massage techniques such as pum-melling and kneading.

Frozen shoulder Light effleurage around the area should help with this because it stimulates the circulation and gets the lymph moving. You can also work on the muscles around the shoulder which will otherwise tend to build up tension.

Headache If this is caused by neck tension, give a neck massage to ease the stiffness. A face and head massage can also help, incorporating massage to the forehead, circling with the thumbs on the temples, and massaging the base of the skull with the fingertips. For a reflexology remedy, try massaging the underside of all your toes apart from the big toe.

See also pp. 156–158.

Indigestion Give a very gentle abdominal massage.

Insomnia See p. 154–156.

Lymphodema This swelling in the arms is caused by trapped lymph fluid as a result of removing the auxiliary lymph nodes during a mastectomy. Firm effleurage in the direction of the shoulder helps, especially with the arm raised.

Period pains Give a slow, deep abdominal massage, allowing your partner to tell you how deeply you can massage.

Rheumatism Gentle massage helps to warm the affected area and stimulates the circulation.

Sciatica This condition causes pain down the centre of the legs at the back, and down the outside of the calf. You can help ease this using light effleurage.

Shoulder tension   A shoulder massage will help, especially if you knead along the top of each shoulder with both hands.

Sinusitis   Give a face massage, and repeat the gliding strokes across the cheeks and around the nose five times.

For a quick sinus treatment, place your thumbs either side of the nostrils and build up the pressure gradually before holding it for about ten seconds.

Sports injuries   See pp. 160–167.

Sprains and strains   These involve damage to ligaments, muscles or tendons. Massage immediately after the injury will help to relieve swelling (but be sure there is no fracture or dislocation first) by helping to drain away the blood and fluid which cause the swelling. Once the injury has healed, deep massage will help to break down any scar tissue.

See also p. 170.

Stiff neck   Kneading on the neck, and working the fingers up the sides of the neck in circling movements, will both help to ease this, as will shoulder massage.

Swollen ankles   These are caused by poor circulation for all sorts of reasons, from insect bites to pregnancy. Use light effleurage from the foot up to the knee, and continue for at least thirty strokes each time you give the treatment.

Tennis elbow   At its worst, this simply needs rest. But when the pain eases, mobilising the joint will help.

Have your partner lie on their back, and hold their arm up so that their hand is towards your stomach. With your partner's palm facing up, support the elbow as you flex it so that the hand moves towards the shoulder. Squeeze the elbow gently as you do this. Repeat this twice, then turn your partner's palm face down and repeat the stretch three more times.

Varicose veins Never massage directly over varicose veins, and don't use petrissage or percussive strokes. However, effleurage around the vein area can help to improve the circulation. Remember always to effleurage up the leg.

INSOMNIA

Which of us hasn't known the horrors, at some time in our life, of not being able to sleep? If we have a partner who suffers from insomnia it may well mean that we suffer too, so learning how to give a massage to counteract this may benefit both partners.

But a massage alone may not be enough – the root causes of persistent and long-term insomnia will also have to be addressed, and this may mean a complete reappraisal of one's lifestyle – especially the stressful elements. There is also quite a lot we can do for ourselves to eliminate other causes of insomnia by establishing a good bedtime routine and avoiding activities and dietary habits that may contribute to sleeplessness.

And if you or your partner still have trouble sleeping you can carry out the following massage before going to bed.

GETTING READY

- As with all massage make sure your partner isn't hungry or too full.

- Any night clothes shouldn't be too tight or so loose they ride up and become uncomfortable.

- Try a warm bath before the massage with a few drops of essential oils – lavender, sandalwood or camomile have all proved to be effective in helping insomnia sufferers.

- Practise the massage over several nights as it may well have a cumulative effect.

- Make sure the bedroom isn't too warm – plenty of fresh air may well be beneficial.

- Make sure the bed itself is firm enough and supports both of you correctly.

---

1 Have your partner lie in the prone position (face down) on the bed and kneel at their head. Lean forward and gently but firmly run your hands down either side of the spine to the lower back. Bring your hands back slowly and very softly. Again push

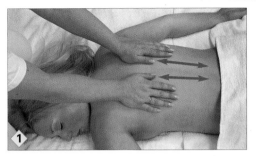

down quite firmly and repeat. Do this several times building up a rhythm of pushing down hard and returning gently. The down stroke should be much slower than the up stroke.

2 Move to their side and begin by kneading the shoulder farthest from you. Slowly work your way down the body kneading all the flesh. Change over to the side nearest you and knead your way back up the body.

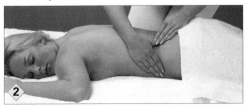

3 Finish by moving back to their head and repeating the up and down strokes either side of their spine six times.

They may well be asleep before you have finished.

HEADACHES

Stopping a headache before it really gets a hold is a skill well worth learning – and identifying the causes of persistent headaches as well. Headaches are the result of the blood vessels at the back of the scalp and neck becoming constricted, leading to contracted muscles in that region. This, in turn, causes tenderness and pain in the back of the head which may often radiate out affecting the temples, eyes and forehead.

This constriction of blood vessels can be brought on by stress, tiredness, worry, eye strain, dietary prob-

---

AVOIDING HEADACHES

- Try to avoid very stressful situations or change your approach to them.

- Eliminate any foods which you know bring on severe headaches or migraines such as chocolate, oranges and red wine.

- If you suffer persistent and painful headaches consult your GP to find out why – and what to do about them.

lems, poor posture – and even atmospheric conditions such as a sudden drop in air pressure.

Once a headache has started the only way to effectively relieve it is to relax those areas affected – the back of the neck, the shoulders and the scalp. Once the muscles are relaxed and the blood vessels returned to normal the pain levels will diminish. A massage to the neck and shoulders will certainly aid in this relaxation process and this is something you can do for yourself. A wet, cold compress applied to your forehead may also help.

At the onset of a headache try the two following massage techniques.

1 If you feel a headache coming on, massage a few drops of diluted lavender oil gently into the temples. Bring your hands up to your head with your fingertips resting lightly on your scalp. Use your thumbs to gently massage your temples. Feel around until you find an exceptionally tender spot and massage that until the headache diminishes.

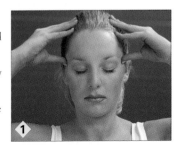

2 At the onset of a headache you can also try massaging the point just above the nose mid-way between your eyebrows. Use your thumb to press quite hard here for a few seconds and release. Press again and release.

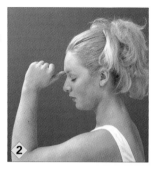

ABDOMINAL COMPLAINTS

Stress affects us all in different ways. It is well known that when we are nervous we experience the feeling of 'butterflies' in the stomach. This is caused by our stomach muscles contracting in case we need to run or stand our ground and fight – the flight or fight reflex. Problems can occur when those muscles fail to relax afterwards. Stress can also cause our digestive tract to produce excessive gastric acid which makes the colon contract abnormally. This in turn presents as the symptoms now known as IBS (Irritable Bowel Syndrome) which can include bloating, excessive wind, diarrhoea, cramps and pain.

So what causes the stress? It can be anger, anxiety, worry, overwork, tension, tiredness, poor diet and poor posture. It can also be brought on by such complaints as pre-menstrual tension. Massage has been proved to be a wonderful natural alleviator of the symptoms of abdominal complaints because it works directly on the areas affected – namely the stomach and colon. Once the muscles have been encouraged to relax the gastric acid returns to normal levels, the food moves through the colon at a better rate – slower in the case of diarrhoea and faster in constipation – the person feels calmer and more tranquil, and pain levels are reduced.

GETTING READY

- Only use very gentle strokes when treating abdominal complaints with massage.

- Don't forget that the digestive tract begins at the mouth and tension can be stored in the jaw – see pp. 96–106 for neck and face massages.

- Always get whoever is being massaged to tell you if they are feeling pain or the pressure you are using is too strong.

- Massage is effective and can replace tranquillisers, pain killers, enemas and laxatives.

- Massage for abdominal complaints may well be cumulative so repeat the massage over several days or weeks.

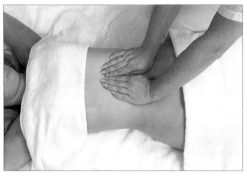

1 Have your partner lie down on their back with their head well supported. Kneel with your knees either side of their legs. Use calm gentle strokes only. Place both hands, one on top of the other, on their navel and push gently upwards towards the chest. Separate your hands and bring them back by letting them glide gently back down the ribs. Repeat this manoeuvre for about ten minutes.

Obviously if in any doubt as to whether a massage should be done check with your GP first to be on the safe side; any other conditions such as persistent constipation or diarrhoea should also be referred.

SPORTS

Sports massage can help sports participants by:

- relieving muscular tension
- speeding recovery of injury
- improving flexibility and mobility
- increasing energy levels
- softening and lengthening muscle fibres
- improving circulation and lymphatic drainage.

GETTING READY

- Always begin with kneading and stroking movements to soften tight muscles and prepare the area for deep pressure work.

- After deep tissue work always use softer massage techniques to restore blood flow to the area

- Check that the person isn't experiencing too much discomfort

- Anyone engaging in sports should exercise for at least twenty minutes two or three times a week

Massage for serious sports injuries calls for a qualified professional, but it's worth looking at other forms of sports massage, including pre- and post-event massage. The best way to avoid injury – especially of the strain and sprain sort – is to be supple and flexible enough in the first place. Pre-event massage can be very important here as it loosens and relaxes the muscles before they are put under undue stress. Post-event massage is beneficial as it loosens muscles that have become too taut due to overexertion.

Any serious injury should be referred to a qualified medical practitioner as soon as possible but if the injury is less serious, such as a strain or sprain or cramp, then there is a lot you can do both for yourself and for others suffering from such complaints.

PRE-EVENT MASSAGE

1 Have your partner lie down in the prone position (face down) and gently knead their entire muscular framework by rhythmically gripping and releasing. This has the effect of encouraging blood flow to the muscles as well as loosening them. Begin at the neck and shoulders and work your way down their back.

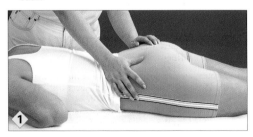

For legs and thighs
see the following
technique.

1 To work on the
thighs and legs
again get them
into the prone
position (face
down) and bend
each leg upwards
at the knee in
turn. Only work
one leg at a time.
Support the
weight of the leg
across your knee
and place your

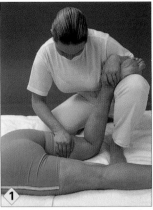

hand on the back of the thigh. Vigorously shake the
muscles of the thigh and release. Lower the leg and
do the same to the calf muscles.

Post-Event Massage

A post-event massage will prevent the onset of muscle
soreness and stiffness.

1 Get your partner to turn over and support your
partner's arm in your hand. Let the arm be as limp
as possible. This enables the lymphatic system to
drain. With your other hand squeeze the arm muscles as firmly as they can tolerate. Squeeze and

POST-EVENT MASSAGE

- Your partner should lie in the prone position (face down, as below).

- Use kneading and rocking movements.

- Use firm pressure on the posterior muscles of the hip as these are prone to tighten after sports and you will restore mobility.

- You can use the weight of your entire body to exert the sort of firm pressure you need to be using.

Post-Event Massage (see above)

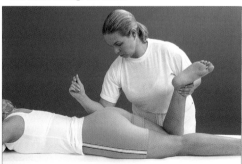

release. Hold their hand and vigorously shake the whole arm. Do the other arm.

2 Keeping them in the same position move slowly around to their head, still holding the arm. Tuck the arm under your armpit and use your other hand to support your partner by placing it along their upper flank. You can now gently pull the arm towards you and release and stretch. This will free up their back muscles – don't overdo it. Do the other arm.

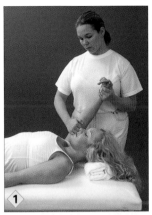

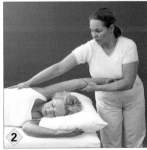

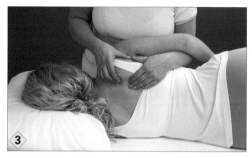

3 Continuing the movement, slowly bring your partner onto their side and cradle the shoulder in your stomach reaching behind them to grip their shoulder blade. Stretch the muscles up towards you and rock the shoulder gently backwards and forwards. Don't use too much pressure on the shoulder blade – get them to tell you if it hurts. Do the other shoulder.

POST-EVENT SELF HELP MASSAGE

To help prevent any post-event muscle stiffness try the following self help massage technique.

1 Sit with your back against a wall or suitable support, reach forward, and grasp the toes of one foot in your hands. Pull the whole foot back towards you and stretch the muscles of the foot and calf. This will improve your post-event flexibility. Stretch and release several times and do the other foot.

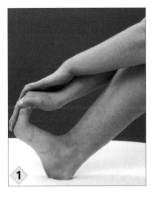

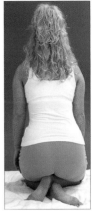

Right: Post-Event Self-Help Massage

POST-EVENT SELF HELP MASSAGE

- Sit back on your legs, kneeling with your ankles crossed. You can put your hands on the floor to help you balance.

- Your body weight alone will stretch the area above your ankles and your calves.

- You can rock backwards and forwards and move your ankles until you feel the stretch working.

CRAMP

Cramp is a static reflex spasm which happens when a muscle has already been shortened and is asked to shorten further. It can be brought on in muscles which have become chronically shortened through excessive use during sport and then have been allowed to atrophy. It can also, it is believed, be caused by low levels of calcium, sodium or glucose in the blood – or even due to dehydration. What we do know is that it is extremely painful and the sudden involuntary contraction of a muscle in spasm that is a cramp can seriously curtail any sporting activity.

If you have access to someone who can massage the cramp you will need deep stroking and kneading of the calves and soles of the feet (*below*), as well as the toe stretching in the previous self help massage.

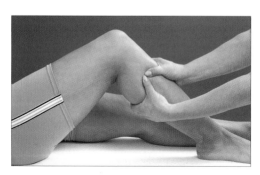

GETTING RID OF CRAMP

Cramp generally affects the calves and feet. Probably the easiest way to get rid of it is to treat the affected area yourself immediately. Sit down with your back against a wall or some other support. Reach forward and, with legs outstretched, grip the toes of the offending leg and stretch the foot towards you as far as it can go (see below). Release and stretch again. Keep this up until the cramp goes.

Someone else may be able to bend your toes much more effectively than you can.

Getting rid of cramp: above

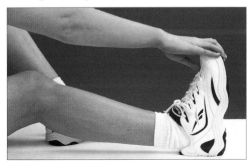

STRAINS AND SPRAINS

A strain is a stretched or torn muscle while a sprain is a twisted or wrenched joint which causes the ligaments to tear and the surrounding tendons and nerves to become damaged.

After the initial pain has worn off, a general massage of the surrounding area can be given to dissipate any tension in the muscles which may have become rigid against the pain. This massage should be gentle but firm to encourage normal muscle action.

DEALING WITH STRAINS AND SPRAINS

First, reduce the inflammation with a cold compress: a wet flannel if there is nothing else, but a pack of frozen vegetables from the freezer is ideal.

Then check that there is nothing broken and massage the area above any swelling. The actual strain or sprain shouldn't be massaged – and will in all probability be far too painful anyway – but gently stroke the adjacent area instead. This causes the blood and fluids surrounding the injury to drain away.

ACHING FEET

Since we walk, on average, around a thousand kilometres a year it's small wonder that we suffer from aching feet – and for athletes and sports people the problem is much worse. The wrong kind of shoes are a big problem for sports fitness; 'trainers' frequently cause excessive sweating, poor circulation and defective ventilation.

Each foot contains 26 bones, thousands of nerve endings and a very delicate network of muscles. Regular massage will alleviate many of the symptoms of tired feet – see pp. 72–77. Problems with the feet will be reflected throughout the entire body so prevention is better than cure – take care of the feet especially if engaged in regular sports.

SELF HELP MASSAGE FOR ACHING FEET

1 Kneel and lean backwards. Clench your fists and place each fist in the sole of your foot. Push upwards and raise your body; the weight transferred to your feet provides excellent massage. You can then use your knuckles to massage the soles of your feet. Keep your weight on the knuckles by pushing

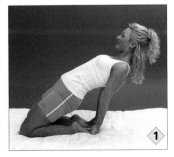

upwards. Rotate the knuckles for a few minutes and then slowly relax.

CARING FOR FEET

- Remove callouses and corns before massaging the feet.

- Soak the feet in lukewarm water and add a few drops of rosemary or lavender oil.

- Massage your feet regularly.

- Always choose well fitting shoes and replace them when worn out.

- Massage the feet gently before sport to warm them up.

RELATED THERAPIES

Shiatsu

This is a Japanese technique which means, translated literally, 'finger pressure'. It is very like acupuncture but instead of using needles on the points, pressure is applied with the fingers and hands.

The belief in China and Japan is that energy, or *chi*, flows through the body along meridians. When this energy becomes blocked or disrupted, it can be restored by applying pressure to the meridians, usually with the thumb or the heel of the hand. Different points along the meridians correspond to different parts of the body, so to treat a particular complaint you would focus on a particular point or meridian – there are about six hundred points in all. However, shiatsu is also a whole body treatment, and is often used simply to rebalance the energy within the body and help prevent illness.

Shiatsu is sometimes reported to be painful, but the pressure applied is not very deep, so it is likely that any pain comes from the blocked *chi* within the point rather than from the nature of the treatment.

PERFORMING SHIATSU

- Shiatsu is a safe and simple therapy to use.

- It requires no equipment.

- It is generally performed on the floor.

- It is done through the clothes.

Shiatsu, like many therapies, is more highly recommended for some conditions than others. To practise it you need to put your body weight into the pressure you apply. So the techniques involve not only knowing where to apply the pressure, but also how to distribute your own weight to make the treatment pleasant and effective for both of you. The illustrations opposite show parallel points where pressure applied can bring particular benefits.

SOME GENERAL POINTS IN SHIATSU: FRONT

1 Headaches

2 Eyes

3 Sinus complaints

4 Tiredness

5 Sickness

7 Stress, insomnia

8 Listlessness

9 PMS (not to be used in pregnancy)

10 Tension, stress

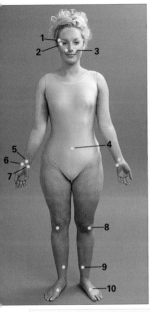
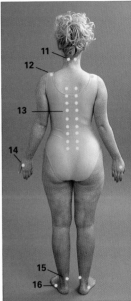

GENERAL POINTS IN SHIATSU: BACK

11 Head, neck, sinus pain

12 Shoulder aches

13 Back complaints

14 Headache (not to be used in pregnancy)

15, 16 Backpain, tiredness

Always apply your weight slowly, and hold the pressure for about five seconds before releasing it and taking your own weight back.

SHIATSU FOR THE BACK

1 With your partner lying on the floor, kneel to one side.

2 Put the heels of your hands on either side of the spine towards the top of the back, with the fingers pointing outwards.

3 Swing your hips forwards to bring your weight to bear on your partner. After five seconds release the pressure and then repeat the movement a little further down the back.

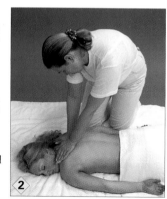

4 When you reach the hips, go back to the beginning again but this time use the thumbs instead of the heel of your hand.

SHIATSU FOR THE BACK OF THE LEGS

1 Get your partner to lie on their stomach with their toes pointed slightly inwards. Kneel beside them facing the legs.

2 Put the hand nearest their back on the far buttock to support yourself (the supporting hand is known in shiatsu as the 'mother hand').

3 Use the palm of the other hand to apply pressure at intervals all down the back of the leg, avoiding the knee.

4 When you reach the heel, squeeze the Achilles tendon in a pinch for about five seconds.

5 Now repeat on the other leg.

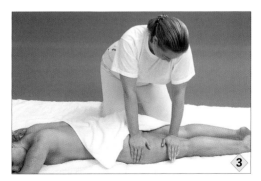

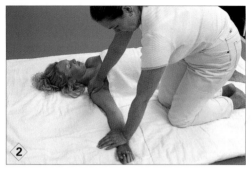

SHIATSU FOR THE ARMS

Your partner needs to lie on their back with the arm you are working on out to the side at a right angle to the body.

1 Kneel alongside the hips, facing the arm; your supporting hand should be around the top of the shoulder.

2 Apply palm pressures down the arm to the wrist with the other hand.

3 Repeat with the other arm.

SHIATSU FOR THE CHEST

1 With your partner lying on their back, kneel with one knee on either side of their head.

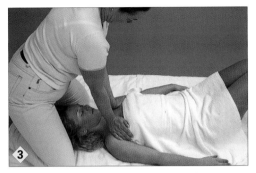

2 Put the heel of each hand in the hollow between the shoulder joint and the collar bone on that side. Your fingers should face outwards.

3 Now bring your hips slowly forward so that your weight is transferred to your hands. Hold this for a few seconds and then release.

4 Now use your palms to make pressures across the chest from the centre to the sides.

5 Finally, use your thumbs to make pressures between the ribs working from the top of the chest down with the thumbs either side of the breastbone.

SHIATSU FOR FATIGUE

1 Have your partner lie on their stomach with their

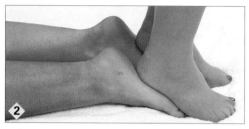

feet about twelve inches apart and resting on a
small cushion.

2 Stand facing away from them, with your weight on
your toes and your heels over their feet.

3 Slowly transfer your weight to your heels, and so
onto their feet.

4 Transfer your weight rhythmically from one foot to
the other by bending each knee in turn.
For deeper pressure, straighten one knee and concentrate on the pressure through that heel.

5 Continue this massage for about ten minutes unless
your partner gets cramp, in which case extend their
big toe and effleurage the instep before returning to
the treatment.

AROMATHERAPY

Aromatherapy is the practice of massage with aromatic

plant oils. These oils can be chosen to increase the effects of the massage, and are especially valuable for releasing emotional tension (*see the A–Z guide on pp. 182–183*). It can be combined with any type of massage, although it is generally used with more superficial movements, so avoiding deep painful, treatments.

The essential oils are too concentrated to be used neat, and should be combined with your carrier oil, at a dilution of about one or two percent. Different oils produce different effects and treat different conditions, so choose an essential oil that is appropriate to the partner you are massaging.

REFLEXOLOGY

This is massage of the feet, which benefits the whole body. It follows the theory that pressure which is applied to specific areas of the feet will affect the organs and systems of the body. It is usually a relaxing, preventative, whole-body treatment, but it can be adapted to focus on any problem part of the body. Its use dates back to the ancient Chinese and Egyptian civilisations, but the system which is generally used today was developed by Dr William H Fitzgerald in 1913. He proposed that the whole body was divided into zones – similar to meridians – which terminated in the feet. Stimulating relevant areas of the foot would therefore influence the parts of the body in that zone.

COMMON ESSENTIAL OILS: AN A–Z

Cypress
Use for: Respiratory problems, rheumatic pains
Warnings: Avoid in the first three months of pregnancy

Eucalyptus
Use for: Pain relief, respiratory problems, stimulant
Warnings: Use low dilution

Frankincense
Use for: Stress

Geranium
Use for: Depression
Warnings: Use low dilution

Ginger
Use for: Warming, stimulating
Warnings: Use low dilution

Jasmine
Use for: Depression, lethargy
Warnings: Avoid during pregnancy and with babies

Juniper
Use for: Aches and pains
Warnings: Avoid during pregnancy

COMMON ESSENTIAL OILS (CONT'D)

Lavender
Use for: Stress, aches and pains, headaches

Neroli
Use for: Stress, depression, emotional stress
Warnings: Use low dilution

Orange
Use for: Depression, lethargy
Warnings: Avoid sunbathing for six hours after use

Peppermint
Use for: Lethargy, headache, digestive problems
Warnings: Use low dilution

Rose
Use for: Depression, stress
Warnings: Use low dilution

Rosemary
Use for: Lethargy, aches and pains
Warnings: Avoid in pregnancy ,with high blood pressure, or epilepsy

Sandalwood
Use for: Stress, skin problems

Ylang ylang
Use for: Depression, stress
Warnings: Use low dilution

To Give a General Reflexology Treatment

Note: Don't use oils or your fingers will tend to slip.

1 Get your partner to sit or lie so that the weight of their leg is supported.

2 Use both hands for the treatment even if one is only giving support at times.

3 Apply pressure with your thumbs, either on a fixed point or by running your thumb along a line of the foot.

4 Use either constant pressure or 'walking' pressure, where you bend and straighten your finger or thumb to move it forwards.

5 Work all over one foot systematically, and then repeat on the other foot.

To Give a Full Reflexology Treatment

For a full reflexology treatment, work your thumb along the various lines of the foot, starting with the diaphragm line just under the ball of the foot, while the other hand supports the top of the foot.

After this, work in the same way on the other main areas of the foot, concentrating on any parts which are tender (indicating troublespots):

Spinal area Apply pressure from the heel of the foot to the big toe, supporting the top of the foot with the other hand.

Head area Work along each toe in turn, from base to tip, beginning with the little toe. Support the toes with the fingers of the same hand, while the other hand supports the top of the foot.

Chest area On the top of the foot, work from the base of each toe to the ankle along the natural furrows.

Digestive area Work in diagonal lines from the waist-line to the diaphragm line, and then from the heel up to the waistline.

Reproductive area Make pressures with your thumb all round the ankle.

Lower back area Make pressures and run the thumb all over the heel.

Finally, complete the treatment for each foot by stroking it gently all over, using a stroking motion towards the toes.

ROLFING

This deep massage technique was developed by Ida Rolf between the 1930s and 1960s. She was a bio-chemist who studied the flexibility of proteins in the connective tissue which holds together the bones, muscles and organs. She believed that muscle tension could be relieved by making this connective tissue more flexible, so this form of massage concentrates on working the connective tissues rather than the muscles.

CONDITIONS ROLFING MAY BENEFIT

- Chronic muscular tension and pain
- Stiff joints
- Poor circulation
- Poor respiration

Rolfing is a deep form of massage, and is often reported to be painful as a result. However, it can bring very fast relief from long-term pain. It is not recommended that untrained practitioners use it, since it calls for a detailed knowledge of anatomy and physiology as well as specific training in rolfing.

HYDROTHERAPY

'Hydrotherapy' means water therapy; every time you put your aching feet in a bowl of warm water – or relax in a hot bath at the end of the day – you are practising hydrotherapy. Taking a cold shower to wake you up is another form of hydrotherapy. The basic principle is that hot water relaxes the muscles by raising your body temperature, while cold water stimulates the circulation and invigorates the skin. You can treat yourself with hydrotherapy, or you can use it to treat someone else.

USING HYDROTHERAPY

There are three ways to use hydrotherapy:

- Using warm water to relax the muscles.

- Using cold water to invigorate and stimulate.

- Alternating hot and cold water to ease cramps or spasms or give an overall workout.

HYDROTHERAPY WORKOUT

For a refreshing, all-over hydrotherapy session:

1 Massage your whole body with a body scrub, using circular movements.

2 Then get into the shower and rinse off.

3 With the shower on hot, and using its most powerful setting, massage all the way up the body from the feet to the neck with small circular movements, spending longest on any areas which feel tense, such as neck and shoulders.

4 Now repeat the hydrotherapy massage with the shower set to cold.

5 Finally, dry off and massage in an invigorating essential oil such as orange.

HYDROTHERAPY FOR CRAMP OR MUSCLE SPASM

You can treat yourself with this method, assuming you can reach the part of your body which is affected. This treatment alternates hot and cold water to relax the muscles and help the circulation.

You will need:

- Two bowls
- Two flannels
- Kettle of boiling water
- Ice cubes

1 Fill one bowl with water as hot as you can stand, and the other with cold water and ice cubes.

What you will need for a hydrotherapy session

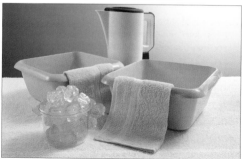

2 Soak a flannel in each bowl.

3 Wring out the hot flannel and hold it against the affected area for thirty seconds.

4 Now return it to the bowl and wring out the cold flannel and hold that in place for thirty seconds.

5 Repeat this half a dozen times; you will probably need to top up the hot water from the kettle or it will cool down too much.

6 At the end of the hydrotherapy, effleurage (*see pp. 14–15*) the area deeply for 30 seconds.

HYDROTHERAPY FOR VARICOSE VEINS

1 Sit in a warm bath with your legs supported out of the water in front of you – resting on the end of the bath will do.

2 Run a cool shower over your leg from the foot up to the knee ten times; repeat with the other leg. (If you don't have a hand shower, a jug of water poured slowly will work.)

3 Empty the bath and dry off your body but not your legs.

4 Wrap your legs in a towel and lie with your lower legs up on a pillow for ten minutes.

FURTHER INFORMATION

USEFUL ADDRESSES

AROMATHERAPY

Aromatherapy Organisations Council
3 Latimer Close
Braybrooke
Market Harborough
Leicester LE16 8LN

International Federation of Aromatherapists
Stamford House
2–4 Chiswick High Road
London W4 1TH
Phone 0181-742 2605

International Society of Professional Aromatherapists
ISPA House
82 Ashby Road
Hinckley
Leicestershire LE10 1SN
Phone 01455-637987

HYDROTHERAPY

UK College of Hydrotherapy
515 Hagley Road
Birmingham B66 4AX
Phone 0121-429 9191

MASSAGE

Massage Therapy Institute of Great Britain
PO Box 276
London NW2 4NR

Massage Training Institute
24 Highbury Road
London
Phone 0171-226 5313

Northern Institute
100 Waterloo Road
Blackpool
Lancashire FY4 1AW
Phone 01253-403548

REFLEXOLOGY

Association of Reflexologists
27 Old Gloucester Street
London WC1N 3XX
Phone 0990-673320

Federation of Precision Reflexologists
38 South Street
Exeter EX1 1ED

International Institute of Reflexology
15 Hartfield Close
Tonbridge
Kent
Phone 01732-350629

SHIATSU

The Shiatsu Society
5 Foxcote, Wokingham
Berkshire
RG11 3PG

FURTHER READING

Massage with Essential Oils
Christine Wildwood (Element 1991)

Manipulation and Mobilisation
Susan L Edmund (Mosby 1993)

Massage and Aromatherapy
Andrew Vickers (Chapman & Hall 1996)

Massage: The Ultimate Illustrated Guide
Clare Maxwell-Hudson (Dorling Kindersley 1999)

Shiatsu: The Complete Guide
C Jarmey and G Mojay (Thorsons 1991)

Teach Yourself Massage
Denise Whichello Brown (Hodder & Stoughton 1996)

The Complete Illustrated Guide to Massage
Stewart Mitchell (Element 1997)

The Complete Illustrated Guide to Reflexology
Inge Dougans (Element 1996)

The Massage Manual Fiona Harrold (Headline 1992)

The Shiatsu Workbook N Dawes (Piatkus 1991)

COLLINS GEM
BABIES' names

COLLINS GEM
BEER

COLLINS GEM
BIRDS

COLLINS GEM
CALORIE Counter

COLLINS GEM
FACT FILE

COLLINS GEM
FENG SHUI

COLLINS GEM
FLAGS

COLLINS GEM
Healthy EATING

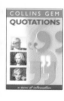

COLLINS GEM
QUOTATIONS

COLLINS GEM
SAS Self-Defence

COLLINS GEM
SAS Survival Guide

COLLINS GEM
SEASHORE

COLLINS GEM
TREES

COLLINS GEM
Understanding DREAMS

COLLINS GEM
WILD flowers

COLLINS GEM
WINE Dictionary